ANNALS OF THE NEW YORK ACADEMY OF SCIENCES

VOLUME 172 ARTICLE 10 PAGES 277–426

January 28, 1971

PHYSIOLOGY AND PATHOLOGY OF TROPHOBLASTIC TUMORS *IN VIVO* AND *IN VITRO* *

CONTENTS

Biological Aspects of Gestational Neoplasms Derived from Trophoblast. *By* ROY HERTZ 279

The Hormone-Synthesizing Trophoblastic Cell *in Vitro:* A Model for Cancer Research and Placental Hormone Synthesis. *By* R. A. PATTILLO, G. O. GEY, E. DELFS, W. Y. HUANG, L. HAUSE, J. GARANCIS, M. KNOTH, J. AMATRUDA, J. BERTINO, H. G. FRIESEN, AND R. F. MATTINGLY 288

The Pathology of Choriocarcinoma. *By* WILLIAM B. OBER, JOHN H. EDGCOMB, and EDWARD B. PRICE, JR. 299

* These papers were presented at a symposium entitled Physiology and Pathology of Trophoblastic Tumors *in Vivo* and *in Vitro,* at a meeting of the Section of Biological and Medical Sciences on October 23, 1969.

Publication of this monograph was aided by contributions from:

- BERNARD G. STEINETZ, Ph.D.
- CIBA PHARMACEUTICAL COMPANY
- HOFFMANN-LaROCHE, INC.
- PRINCETON LABORATORIES
- THE SCHERING CORPORATION
- SMITH KLINE AND FRENCH LABORATORIES
- THE SQUIBB INSTITUTE FOR MEDICAL RESEARCH
- WARNER-LAMBERT RESEARCH INSTITUTE

BIOLOGICAL ASPECTS OF GESTATIONAL NEOPLASMS DERIVED FROM TROPHOBLAST

Roy Hertz, M.D., Ph.D.

The Population Council
Rockefeller University
New York, N.Y.

Introduction

This report will describe certain features of the biological behavior of tumors derived from trophoblast either during or after pregnancy in women. These tumors are termed "gestational trophoblastic neoplasms" in order to distinguish them from such trophoblast-containing tumors as embryonal carcinomas arising in the testes, ovaries, or other sites. These latter tumors are referred to collectively as "non-gestational trophoblastic neoplasms."[1] Our conclusions regarding the nature and behavior of gestational trophoblastic neoplasms stem from direct clinical and laboratory observation of over three hundred instances of this type of tumor over the past two decades. Two hundred of these cases represented "metastatic trophoblastic neoplasms," a term used to indicate that the disease had spread beyond the uterus. The remainder were instances of "non-metastatic trophoblastic neoplasms," with the disease limited to the uterine fundus.[2]

Classical morphologists have regarded gestational neoplasms as including three distinct entities that can be readily separated on histopathological grounds.[3] Hence, these tumors are usually considered to comprise (*a*) hydatidiform mole, (*b*) chorioadenoma destruens (invasive mole), and (*c*) choriocarcinoma. The distinguishing feature of these entities is the degree of retention of recognizable villous structures in the neoplastic chorionic tissue. Hence, in those instances in which the entire tumor mass is confined to the uterine cavity and is made up of hydatidiform villi with limited trophoblastic overgrowth, the lesion is termed a "hydatidiform mole." Whenever the tumor has invaded the uterine wall or extrauterine tissues but retains residual villous structures, it is termed an "invasive mole" or "chorioadenoma destruens." In the absence of any residual villous structures, a gestational trophoblastic tumor further characterized by invasiveness, hemorrhage, and necrosis is termed a "choriocarcinoma." Despite these clearly defined morphological criteria, a vast amount of confusion arises in daily clinical practice with respect to the diagnostic and, particularly, the prognostic significance of these purely structural terms. Nevertheless, over 50% of patients with what ultimately becomes a "choriocarcinoma" have a clear history of having previously had a "hydatidiform mole," and numerous patients with a prior histological diagnosis of "invasive mole" subsequently present tissue clearly characteristic of "choriocarcinoma." We have, therefore, inferred that these tumors constitute a biological continuum, each merging imperceptibly into the other. The situation is further complicated by the fact that the maternal host possesses an inherent capability of rejecting the invading fetal tissue, thus leading to rare but well-documented spontaneous regression of the tumor process associated with complete absence of residual disease in some cases.[4] Accordingly, any prognostic inferences or any therapeutic claims in relation to gestational trophoblastic tumors must involve a large number of cases carefully evaluated on both clinical and morphological grounds, and with a full appreciation of the highly varied and complex dynamic interrelationship between these several forms of tumor.

Biological Classification

It would be inappropriate to detail our clinical experience with the chemotherapy of choriocarcinoma and related trophoblastic tumors in women in this paper, since these purely clinical observations are available elsewhere.[2,5] However, certain aspects of our chemotherapeutic experience have aided us in the biological characterization of these tumor processes. Table 1 summarizes our therapeutic results in 113 cases of metastatic trophoblastic disease in relation to the duration of disease prior to treatment. It is clear that a much higher remission rate is obtained in patients with a brief disease history than in those with a prolonged illness. This increasing resistance to the elimination of all trophoblastic tissue suggests that a progressive adaptation between tumor and host tissue occurs with time. This mutual adaptation between host and tumor tissue of differing genetic constitution may be interpreted as indicating either a lack of immunogenic potential on the part of the invading trophoblast or special instances of failure of such an immune mechanism. However, we have now observed 70 subsequent pregnancies in women previously freed by chemotherapy of even extensive metastatic trophoblastic disease. Thus, the massive infiltration of the lungs and other peripheral tissues with highly proliferative malignant trophoblast fails to impart any resistance to the subsequent tolerance to the intrauterine growth of normal trophoblastic elements. In one instance, a normal pregnancy occurred within 3 months of the subsidence of the trophoblastic disease process. It would seem, therefore, that if any immune response had occurred, it would have had to be short-lived.

Table 1
Influence of Duration of Disease on Outcome

Duration of Disease (months)	Complete Remissions (total no. of patients)	
	Series A	Series B
4 or less	18/25 (72%)	23/27 (85%)
4 or more	12/38 (31%)	14/23 (61%)
Totals	30/63 (48%)	37/50 (74%)

Alternatively, one is obliged to consider the intrauterine environment as a special locus for such tolerance. Paradoxically, malignant trophoblast has extreme difficulty in surviving for any length of time in the uterine cavity. This is attested to by the almost uniform absence of tumor within the uterus at autopsy in untreated women dying with extensive metastatic disease. In thirty autopsies on previously treated women we have found no instance of intrauterine disease.

This frequent subsidence of the primary tumor focus despite metastatic tumor dissemination is a unique phenomenon among all malignancies. It is also especially noteworthy that intramural masses of tumor within the uterine wall are, on the contrary, very resistant to chemotherapy.[2]

The functional comparison of malignant and normal trophoblastic tissue reveals many similarities and a few differences. Both malignant and normal trophoblast are highly proliferative and extremely vascular. The growth rate and mitotic index of both are very high. Each proliferates a vast endothelial bed permitting an enormous blood flow. This feature manifests itself clinically in a marked predisposition to massive and intractable hemorrhage in patients with metastatic trophoblastic neoplasms.

The most prominent hormonal feature of both normal and malignant trophoblast is the production of chorionic gonadotropin. Because of the astronomically high titers of chorionic gonadotropin seen in some patients with relatively limited extent of disease, the question of identifying tumor hormone with normal pregnancy hormone has been raised. Accordingly, we undertook to compare the fractional distribution of chorionic gonadotropin in the plasma of 12 normally pregnant women and 12 women with metastatic choriocarcinoma. We found that although hormonal activity is found in the γ- and β-globulin fractions in normal pregnancy, this activity is found mainly in the α-globulin fraction in women with choriocarcinoma. This finding is interpreted as representing a difference in hormone transport rather than any significant difference in chemical composition of the chorionic hormone in the normal and neoplastic state.[6] This interpretation is strengthened by our finding that the dose-response curve for the ovarian-weight response in the rat is identical for hormone prepared from the urine of tumor-bearing women and that of normally pregnant women. Moreover, despite extensive attempts to differentiate immunologically between tumor hormone and pregnancy hormone, we have been unable to detect any significant difference as manifested by comparative behavior in Ouchterlony plates, dose-response curves of respective antisera in bioassay systems, or in red-cell agglutination-inhibition tests of antisera to each type of hormone. It is therefore our present interpretation that tumor hormone and pregnancy hormone are very similar, and probably identical.

Nevertheless, the unusually high titers seen in some cases suggest that an especially potent form of the hormone may be arising from malignant trophoblast. Conversely, it is noteworthy that most patients who exhibit resistance to chemotherapy, after an initial marked but incomplete regression of disease, maintain a relatively uniform level of residual urinary gonadotropin titer, usually 250–500 international units (IU) per 24 hours. The constancy of this finding in 20 out of 28 such cases studied suggests either that the chemotherapeutically resistant cells may be producing an atypical form of chorionic hormone or that they have a limited capacity to produce biologically active substance.

An equally puzzling phenomenon observed in the ovaries of tumor-bearing women merits discussion. In about one-third of women with recently developed trophoblastic neoplasms there is a massive enlargement of the ovaries. Such enlarged ovaries consist of huge follicles, corpora hemorrhagica, and corpora lutea. Endocrinologically, this is interpreted as representing the result of a synergistic gonadotropic effect of endogenous pituitary and chorionic gonadotropin. Paradoxically, as the disease process advances, and despite great increments in urinary and plasma levels of chorionic gonadotropin, the ovaries involute rapidly so that within 4 months they are of normal size as observed clinically and at autopsy. Moreover, such ovaries then present an entirely normal histological appearance, with no residual evidence of their previous stimulation. This refractoriness to further gonadotropic stimulation may reflect the failure of continued production of endogenous pituitary hormone required for synergistic action with the ever-increasing amounts of tumor chorionic hormone. An additional phenomenon of endocrine interest is the reestablishment of normal, cyclic vaginal bleeding, despite the persistence of the low residual chorionic hormone titers in women in incomplete remission. In such cases, the ovary appears to be responding to cyclic endogenous pituitary function without being affected by the reduced chorionic gonadotropin.

The occurrence of hyperthyroidism in women with trophoblastic disease has been noted for some time. Since both of these diseases occur somewhat selectively in young women, it has been difficult to determine whether their simultaneous occurrence can be attributed to coincidence. In our experience with 93 patients with metastatic trophoblastic disease in whom the customary parameters of thyroid function were studied, we encountered seven women with laboratory evidence of increased thyroid function. Assay of tumor tissue from two of these patients revealed the presence of thyroid-stimulating hormone (thyrotropin, TSH) in amounts greatly exceeding that found in blood. In two other patients, elevated plasma levels of TSH were demonstrable. Moreover, in these patients the suppression of the disease by the folic acid antagonist methotrexate was accompanied by a prompt return of their thyroid-function test results to normal without specific antithyroid therapy. Hence, it would appear that certain trophoblastic tumors produce thyrotropin as well as gonadotropin.[7]

The development of an accurate and specific radioimmunoassay for human placental lactogen (HPL) has permitted the determination of the comparative plasma levels of this hormone in normal pregnant women and in women with trophoblastic tumors. Whereas there is a progressive increment in the plasma level of HPL during the course of normal pregnancy, the initially low plasma level of HPL in tumor-bearing women fails to rise with time. This discrepancy is thought by some to provide a basis for a good differential diagnostic test between these two conditions.[8,9]

Patients with hydatidiform mole frequently exhibit a striking toxemia-like syndrome. This consists of hypertension, edema, albuminuria, and hyperemesis. All of these features subside promptly when the mole is removed. The humoral basis for this syndrome is yet to be elucidated, but a derangement in steroid metabolism is suggested by the clinical findings.

Animal Studies

It was Greene who initially described the survival and growth of human malignant tissue in the anterior chamber of the guinea pig eye.[10] These pioneer studies provided the basic experimental background for the observations reported in this paper. Subsequently, Toolan[11] and Sommers and his colleagues[12] introduced the use of the hamster cheek pouch as a site for such heterologous tumor transfer. They also found that the frequency of tumor "takes" could be significantly increased by suppression of the immune response of the host animal prior to tumor transplantation. This was accomplished through x-irradiation or cortisone administration or through a combination of both of these procedures. Pierce and co-workers[13] showed that certain human testicular tumors could be maintained as heterologous grafts by serial passage through similarly conditioned hamsters. They found that such tumors continued to produce the chorionic type of gonadotropin even after prolonged maintenance in the foreign host.

In our studies, tumor tissue was initially obtained under aseptic conditions within 1–7 hours after surgical excision or necropsy (TABLE 2). Female golden hamsters of the National Institutes of Health (NIH) strain varying from 1 to 3 months in age were employed. Purina checkers were fed as a basal diet, and a daily ration of kale, apples, and carrots was provided. Under sodium pentobarbital (Nembutal®) anesthesia, each hamster received by direct inoculation into the cheek pouch a piece of freshly excised tissue, about 0.05 cc in volume. Recipient hamsters were either left totally untreated or received 3 mg of cortisone acetate in aqueous suspension at the time of inoculation and every third day for the ensuing 2 weeks. Repeated inspection of the everted cheek pouch revealed the course of growth of the tumor inocula, and this was recorded by a freehand sketch of the size and shape of the growing tumor mass. Histological studies were performed on certain specimens after fixation in Bouin's solution and staining with hematoxylin and eosin. Hamster plasma was prepared from heparinized blood drawn from the abdominal aorta under pentobarbital anesthesia just prior to autopsy. Detailed observations were recorded at autopsy

TABLE 2

SEVEN STRAINS OF HUMAN CHORIOCARCINOMA IN HAMSTER CHEEK POUCH

Strain	Date Started	Source†	Clinical Status of Patient
BO	7/22/57	Metastasis to breast (S)	Incomplete remission on MTX; cerebral hemorrhage while off therapy; strain requires cortisone
WO	10/24/58	Brain metastasis (A)	Resistant to MTX after initial response
MA	11/12/58	Lung metastasis (A)	Resistant to MTX after initial response
JO	11/11/59	Lung metastasis	Resistant to MTX after initial response; then no response to VLB or Cytoxan®
RE	1/21/60	Metastasis to cervix (S)	No chemotherapy before tissue obtained; subsequent complete remission on MTX followed by actinomycin D, although still potentially responsive to MTX
GR	11/2/60	Brain metastasis (A)	Limited response to MTX and VLB, followed by resistance to both drugs
CA	9/26/61	Lung metastasis (A)	No initial response to MTX or actinomycin D

*All hamsters were treated daily via subcutaneous injection, beginning on day 6 after transplantation of the tumor strain; effective doses of the drugs used were: 50 mg/kg for methotrexate (MTX), 0.75 mg/kg for vinblastine (VBL), and 50 μg/kg for actinomycin D.

†Source of tumor strain: S = surgical specimen, A = autopsy.

concerning the qualitative and quantitative effects of the tumor transplant on various endocrine organs.

All chemotherapeutic agents were administered daily, subcutaneously, in the form and dosage indicated in TABLE 2. The drugs were all started on day 6 after transplantation, when initial growth of the transplant could be clearly observed. Repeated sketches of the size and form of the tumors of treated and untreated control animals provided an estimate of the extent of inhibitory effects obtained.

Upon discontinuing serial passage of each strain, portions of tumor were preserved in 50% saline and 50% glycerol under liquid-nitrogen refrigeration. The frozen tissue from each strain was subsequently successfully reinoculated into untreated hamsters whenever further study was required. The seven successfully established strains of choriocarcinoma resulted from a total of thirty attempts. Five of these strains "took" initially in totally untreated hamsters, and all but one strain can be maintained in such untreated animals. Cortisone conditioning has been continuously required for the transfer of one strain even after extended passage over a period of 12 years. However, this strain differs in no other observable feature from those maintained without cortisone.

The growth behavior is essentially the same for all seven strains. The initial host response consists of the appearance of a turbid exudate about the tumor inoculum within 2–3 days. In the following 3 days, this is rapidly replaced by highly vascularized, bluish-purple tissue that then extends and rapidly fills the cheek pouch. In about 10–12 days, the tumor reaches its maximum size of 1–1.5 cc. During the ensuing 5–10 days, the tumor loses its bluish color and becomes successively pink, gray, and finally greenish-yellow. At this point the necrotizing mass may slough and drain. Frequently, only a small residual scar may be found in the cheek pouch by 30 days following inoculation. Less frequently, the liquefied tumor mass is indefinitely retained. Within 10–14 days after inoculation, about 90% of the takes are observed, and 60–80% of the takes are apparent after the first 6 days. These findings are the same for previously frozen tissue.

Histological study of all strains reveals a close similarity between the morphology of the transplant and that seen in the original human material. The rich vascularity of the tumor is very striking, the vascular elements and extravasated blood constituting about one-half of the tumor mass. Both cytotrophoblast and syncytiotrophoblast are clearly distinguishable, although in some preparations the syncytiotrophoblast is scant. It is noteworthy that although this heterologously maintained tissue derives from tumor that is highly invasive in its natural host, no evidence of invasion of surrounding host tissue is observed in the hamster cheek pouch. In addition, whether the tumor is implanted subcutaneously, intraperitoneally, or intracerebrally, it grows at the site of implantation but has never been observed to invade or metastasize in a single one of the thousands of animals observed. The application of massive cortisone dosage has not altered its behavior in this regard.

Galton and his associates[14] have described the chromosomal makeup of one of our tumor strains. The tumor is stated to "reveal an unstable and individually variable aneuploid karyotype. The modal chromosome number at the 56th passage was 80, and, after an interval of 9 months, at the 80th generation, it had risen to 88–92. However, there was no concomitant change in tumor histology." Wynn and Davies[15] have described the ultrastructure of this same tumor strain. Electron microscopy revealed cells resembling normal syncytiotrophoblast in that the cytoplasm contained abundant endocytoplasmic reticulum, ribosomes, and distinctive Golgi bodies. Distinctly cytotrophoblastic cells were also identified, and a type of transitional cell was described with structural resemblance in some features to both cytotrophoblast and syncytiotrophoblast.

Of major interest is the sustained hormonal activity of all of our tumor strains. From what is known of hormonal production by normal trophoblastic tissue, the primary hormone to be expected would be chorionic gonadotropin. In addition, thyrotropin might be expected in view of the demonstrated association of hyperthyriodism with malignant trophoblastic disease, and its suppression by oncolytic chemotherapy, as well as the presence of excessive quantities of thyrotropin in the human plasma and tumor, as demonstrated by bioassay. Finally, the possible presence of HPL, as noted previously, must be considered in view of the frequency of persistent lactation in women with trophoblastic disease.

The intact female hamster bearing any of our tumor strains exhibits an extreme gonadotropic response consisting initially of extensive follicular stimulation, which subsequently gives way to extensive luteinization. Although hemorrhagic follicles are frequently seen, ovulation is not observed. The uterus shows marked enlargement and hyperemia, reflecting the ovarian hormonal response. These ovarian and uterine effects are seen in essentially the same degree in the hypophysectomized tumor-bearing hamster. However, no uterine effects are observed in the ovariectomized hamster, indicating a lack of steroid-type hormone production.

The mammary glands of the intact tumor-bearing hamster are not grossly stimulated. However, detailed microscopical examination of such mammary tissue has not been carried out. Immunofluorescence study of the tumor tissue is also indicated, since Sciarra and co-workers[16] have demonstrated the presence of a "growth hormone-prolactin" in normal syncytiotrophoblast through the application of specific fluoresceinized antiserum. In the hypophysectomized hamster, there is neither gross nor histological evidence of thyrotrophic effect or adrenocorticotrophic effect from the tumor. These negative observations apply equally to all strains, despite the fact that the CA strain was derived at autopsy from a patient who had been freed of prior evidence of hyperthyroidism by oncolytic therapy.[7]

The distribution of the tumor-produced gonadotropin in the host's tissues has been repeatedly studied for several strains by means of bioassay of body fluids or tissue homogenates by either the rat ovarian-weight assay or the mouse uterine-weight assay. Fresh tumor homogenates contain about 50 IU/g. Urine and blood contains about 20–30 IU/ml. It is, however, interesting that homogenates of liver, kidney, muscle, and spleen contain no detectable biological activity. This indicates that although the hormone can be cleared by the kidney, it does not readily enter the cells of peripheral tissues.

The ultimate rejection of the tumor by the host indicates a delayed immune response to the presence of heterologous tissue. Accordingly, we have found that a hamster which has previously rejected a tumor after several weeks of growth is completely resistant to reinoculation for at least several months. Moreover, the daily injection of 2 ml of plasma from such a tumor-resistant animal will completely inhibit tumor growth in a previously untreated hamster. Hence, both active and passive resistance to tumor inoculation may be demonstrated. However, prior exposure of hamsters to human serum globulin will also impart such resistance to tumor inoculation. This indicates that the resistance relates to the formation of species-specific antibodies against antigens of human origin and not to tumor-specific antigens. This phase of induced resistance to tumor inoculation merits extensive study.

Another immunological aspect of these studies relates to the fact that chorionic gonadotropin is known to be specifically antigenic in numerous species.

Antibodies to this hormonal antigen can be readily demonstrated by classical immunological methods as well as by neutralization of hormonal effects in bioassay. Accordingly, we have tested by bioassay the sera of animals having previously borne hormone-producing choriocarcinoma for evidence of anti-hormonal activity. In no instance was such anti-hormonal activity demonstrable. Moreover, prolonged administration of massive doses of purified human chorionic gonadotropin to normal hamsters failed to yield anti-hormonal sera. Accordingly, it would seem that although the hamster shows good immune response to growing human choriocarcinoma as well as to human serum globulin, chorionic gonadotropin is not an effective antigen in this species.

The effects of a wide variety of drugs upon the growth of well-established tumors during the second week following inoculation have been studied according to procedures outlined previously. Our most extensive work has been with methotrexate. We were impressed at the outset by the remarkably high tolerance of the hamster for methotrexate. Such unusual resistance to the effect of colchicine had been previously described.[17] Similarly, we found that the required dose for complete tumor inhibition was about 50 mg/kg, administered subcutaneously on each of 4 consecutive days (TABLE 2). This represents about 100 times the dose found to induce clinical toxicity and tumor response in women. Nevertheless, in the hamster this very high dosage produced no apparent systemic toxicity, normally manifested by loss of body weight, change in coat quality, diarrhea, or ulceration of oral mucous membranes.

Profound tumor inhibition was uniformly observed in all seven strains of tumor in response to this dose of methotrexate. It should be emphasized that five of these strains originated from patients who had exhibited unequivocal evidence of unresponsiveness to previously effective doses of methotrexate (TABLE 2). This discrepancy may rest on the fact that in the experimental system we are testing the growth and survival of freshly transplanted tumor cells from a heterologous source, whereas in the patient these same tumor cells are isologous and have been resident in the host for prolonged periods by the time drug resistance is encountered. The quantitative difference in tolerated dosage between human and hamster is probably not a factor in the discrepancy, inasmuch as the effective dose of other drugs tested is comparable in human and hamster despite similar discrepancies between drug responsiveness shown by two species. This, then, is a good demonstration of the great fallibility of considering animal experimental data to be directly applicable to man.

We have previously described the marked suppression of growth of these tumor strains produced by the *Vinca* alkaloids.[18] In the case of vinblastine, the effective and well-tolerated dose in the hamster closely approximated the effective but highly toxic dose in women.[19] Moreover, this drug was effective in two strains of tumor derived from patients in whom a prior therapeutic trial had induced no apparent tumor response. Actinomycin D has similarly proven uniformly effective in inhibiting all seven tumor strains, although one of these was derived from a patient who had proven totally unresponsive to this compound (TABLE 2).

In addition to the aforementioned drugs, we have screened a wide variety of steroidal, alkaloidal, and antibiotic preparations for possible inhibitory effect. The only significant inhibition observed not related to general systemic toxicity has been in the case of such alkylating agents as cyclophosphamide and in several preparations derived from podophyllotoxin. The activity observed in this latter group of agents warrants further investigation with a view to possible clinical trial.

References

1. Holland, J. F. & M. M. Hreshchyshyn. 1967. Choriocarcinoma. Unio Int. Contra Cancrum. Monograph Series. Vol. **3**: Appendix I. Springer-Verlag. Berlin, Germany.
2. Hertz, R. 1968. Eigenschaften und Behandlung des Choriokarzinoms und verwandter Trophoblast-Tumoren bei Frauen. Geburtsh. Frauenheilk. **28**: 810–823.
3. Novak, E. & C. S. Seah. 1954. Choriocarcinoma of the uterus: Study of 74 cases from Matthieu Registry. Amer. J. Obstet. Gynec. **67**: 933–961.
4. Brewer, J. I. 1961 Textbook of Gynecology. 3rd edit. The Williams & Wilkins Co. Baltimore, Md.
5. Ross, G. T., D. P. Goldstein, R. Hertz, M. B. Lipsett & W. D. Odell. 1965. Sequential use of methotrexate and actinomycin D in the treatment of metastatic choriocarcinoma and related trophoblastic disease. Amer. J. Obstet Gynec. **93**: 223–229.
6. Reisfeld, R. A., D. M. Bergenstal & R. Hertz. 1959. Distribution of gonadotropic hormone activity in the serum proteins of normal pregnant women and patients with trophoblastic tumors. Arch. Biochem. **81**: 456–463.
7. Odell, W. D., R. W. Bates, R. S. Rivlin, M. B. Lipsett & R. Hertz. 1963. Increased thyroid funstion without clinical hyperthyroidism in patients with choriocarcinoma. J. Clin. Endocr. **23**: 658–664.
8. Saxena, B. 1967. Serum placental lactogen levels in trophoblastic diseases. Transcript 4th Rochester Trophoblastic Cont. : 423–438. Rochester University Publ. Rochester, N.Y.
9. Josimovich, J. B. & J. A. MacLaren. 1962. Presence in the human placenta and term serum of a highly lactogenic substance immunologically related to pituitary growth hormone. Endocrinology **71**: 209–220.
10. Greene, H. S. N. 1952. The significance of the heterologous transplant ability of human cancer. Cancer **5**: 24–44.
11. Toolan, H. W. 1953. Growth of human tumors in cortisone-treated laboratory animals: The possibility of obtaining permanently transplantable human tumors. Cancer Res. **13**: 389–394.
12. Sommers, S. C., R. N. Chute & S. Warren. 1952. Heterotransplantation of human cancer. I. Irradiated rats. Cancer Res. **12**: 909–911.
13. Pierce, B., E. L. Berney & F. J. Dixon. 1957. The biology of testicular cancer. I. Behavior after transplantation. Cancer Res. **17**: 134–138.
14. Galton, M., P. B. Goldman & S. Holt. 1963. Karyotypic and morphologic characteristization of a serially transplanted human choriocarcinoma. J. Nat. Cancer Inst. **31**: 1019–1035.
15. Wynn, R. M. & J. Davies. 1964. Ultrastructure of transplanted choriocarcinoma and its endocrine implications. Amer. J. Obstet. Gynec. **88**: 618–633.
16. Sciarra, J. J., S. J. Kaplan & M. M. Grumbach. 1963. Localization of antihuman growth hormone serum within the human placenta; evidence for a human chorionic growth hormone prolactin. Nature **199**: 1005–1006.
17. Orsini, M. W. & B. Paustry. 1952. The natural resistance of the golden hamster to colchicine. Science **115**: 88–89.
18. Hertz, R. 1960. Suppression of human choriocarcinoma maintained in the hamster cheek-pouch by extracts and alkaloids of *Vinca rosea*. Proc. Soc. Exp. Biol. Med. **105**: 281–282.
19. Hertz, R., M. B. Lipsett & R. H. Moy. 1960. Effect of cincaleukoblastine on metastatic choriocarcinoma and related trophoblastic tumors in women. Cancer Res. **20**: 1050–1053.

THE HORMONE-SYNTHESIZING TROPHOBLASTIC CELL *IN VITRO:* A MODEL FOR CANCER RESEARCH AND PLACENTAL HORMONE SYNTHESIS

R. A. Pattillo, M.D., G. O. Gey, M. D.,* E. Delfs, M. D.,
W. Y. Huang, Ph.D., L. Hause, Ph.D, J. Garancis, M.D.,
M. Knoth, M.D.,† J. Amatruda, M.D., J. Bertino, M.D.,‡
H. G. Friesen, M.D.,§ and R. F. Mattingly, M.D.

Medical College of Wisconsin, Milwaukee, Wis.

The human trophoblast, the hormonally functional cell of the placenta, differentiates in the first-order cleavage of the fertilized human ovum immediately following conception.[1] Hormonal function from the placental trophoblast can be detected in maternal serum by human chorionic gonadotropin (HCG)[2] and human placental lactogen (HPL)[3] assays shortly following the 58-cell stage of the human ovum. Thus, trophoblastic cellular differentiation and placental hormone synthesis are among the earliest morphological and biochemical differentiations to occur in the human. This cell type has not been established *in vitro.*

Choriocarcinoma is a unique malignancy of trophoblastic cells which follows normal pregnancy, spontaneous abortion, or hydatiform mole. This tumor closely parallels the normal placenta in hormone function and cellular metabolism, with the exception that the limited invasiveness of the normal placenta during its implantation is far exceeded by that of the malignant tumor, which, proceeding unrestricted, culminates in the death of the patient within a period of less than 1 year.[4] A morphological similarity can be observed among the trophoblastic cells of the human blastocyst less than 92 hours after conception (FIGURE 1), the invading normal placenta of the first trimester (FIGURE 2), and the rapidly proliferating choriocarcinoma (FIGURE 3).

Trophoblast Cell Model

Using a continuous line of trophoblastic cells from human choriocarcinoma, a series of investigations of cancer cell properties and placental hormone synthesis have been initiated in the various institutions contributing to this report. The original choriocarcinoma specimen was successfully established by serial transplantation in the hamster cheek pouch by Hertz.[5] Using this specimen, Pattillo and Gey established the first continuous human hormone-synthesizing tissue in cell culture[6] in 1966; this tissue has maintained stable growth characteristics, with production of the multiple placental hormones characteristic of normal pregnancy.

*Johns Hopkins Medical Institution, Baltimore, Md.
†Reproductive Biology Laboratory, Rigshospitalet, Copenhagen, Denmark.
‡Yale University School of Medicine, New Haven, Conn.
§McGill University, Montreal, Canada.

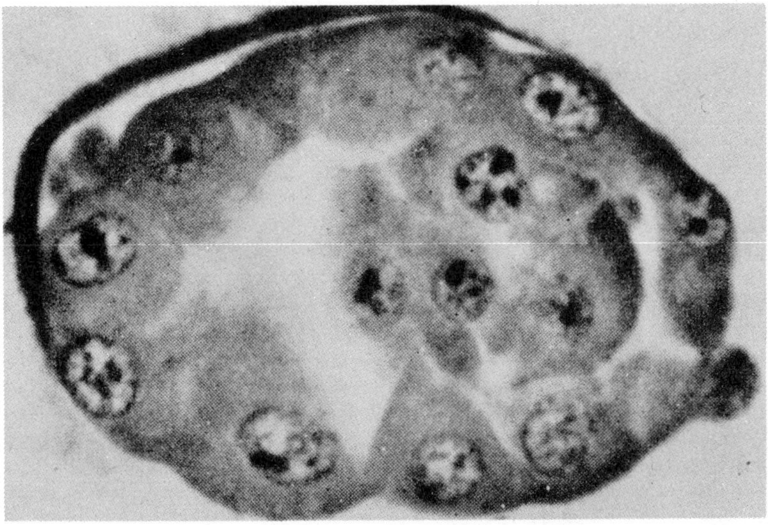

FIGURE 1. A 58-cell blastocyst. The peripheral trophoblast cells make up the bulk of the conceptus less than 92 hours after the first cell division. (× 600) From Hertig.[1]

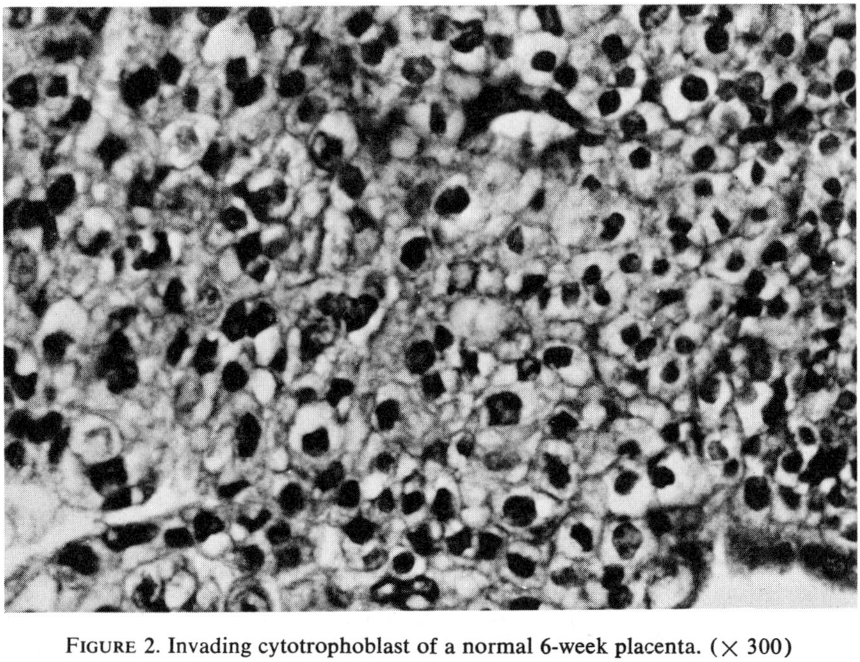

FIGURE 2. Invading cytotrophoblast of a normal 6-week placenta. (× 300)

The morphology of this cell line in continuous culture is shown under light microscopy in FIGURE 3. Under electron microscopy, the organelle structure of the cytotrophoblast is demontrated (FIGURE 4). Intermediate differentiation in

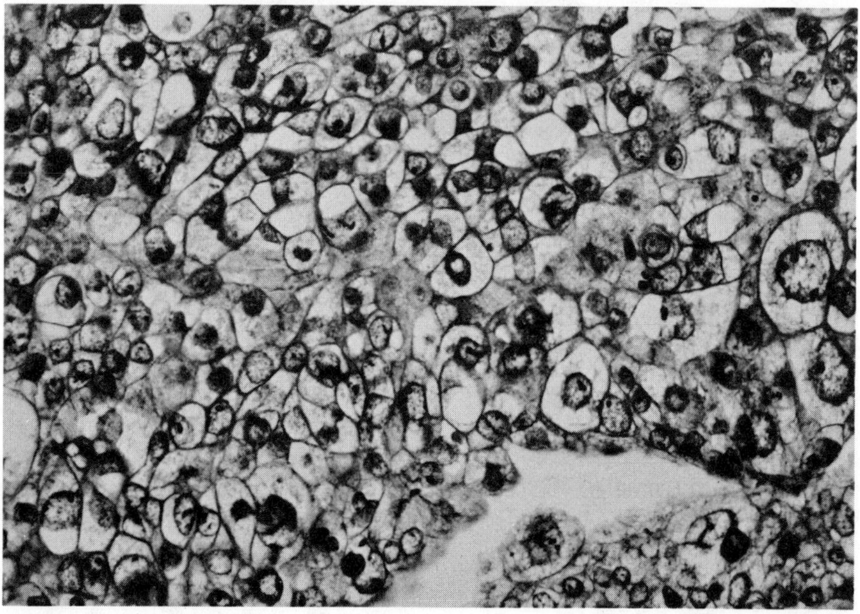

FIGURE 3. A PAS-digested section of the BeWo trophoblast cells from a tissue-culture flask. (× 300)

FIGURE 4. Electron micrograph of a BeWo trophoblast cell from a culture flask, showing heavy glycogen (GL) content; note the prominent desmosomes, Golgi apparatus, and lysosomes (L). N = nucleus; M = mitochondrion. (× 10,000)

the cytotrophoblast is observed. Many desmosomes are present, illustrating the unicellular characteristics of the cytotrophoblast, in contrast to the differentiated synctio-trophoblast, which only abortively forms and does not remain viable in the rapidly growing culture. There is an active Golgi apparatus, and the mitochondria show apparent normal structure. Prominent lysosomes are present, and glycogen concentration is notable, the intensity of which varies according to the concentration of glucose in the culture medium.

HUMAN CHORIONIC GONADOTROPIN SYNTHESIS

Human chorionic gonadotropin (HCG), the most fundamental hormone of the cytotrophoblast, critical in maintaining function of the corpus luteum and in stimulating steroid biosynthesis,[7] is commonly used in bio- and immunoassays to diagnose normal pregnancy and to monitor the treatment of trophoblastic tumors, which continue to secrete the characteristic hormone in large quantities. This hormone was used as a functional marker for identification of the tropho-

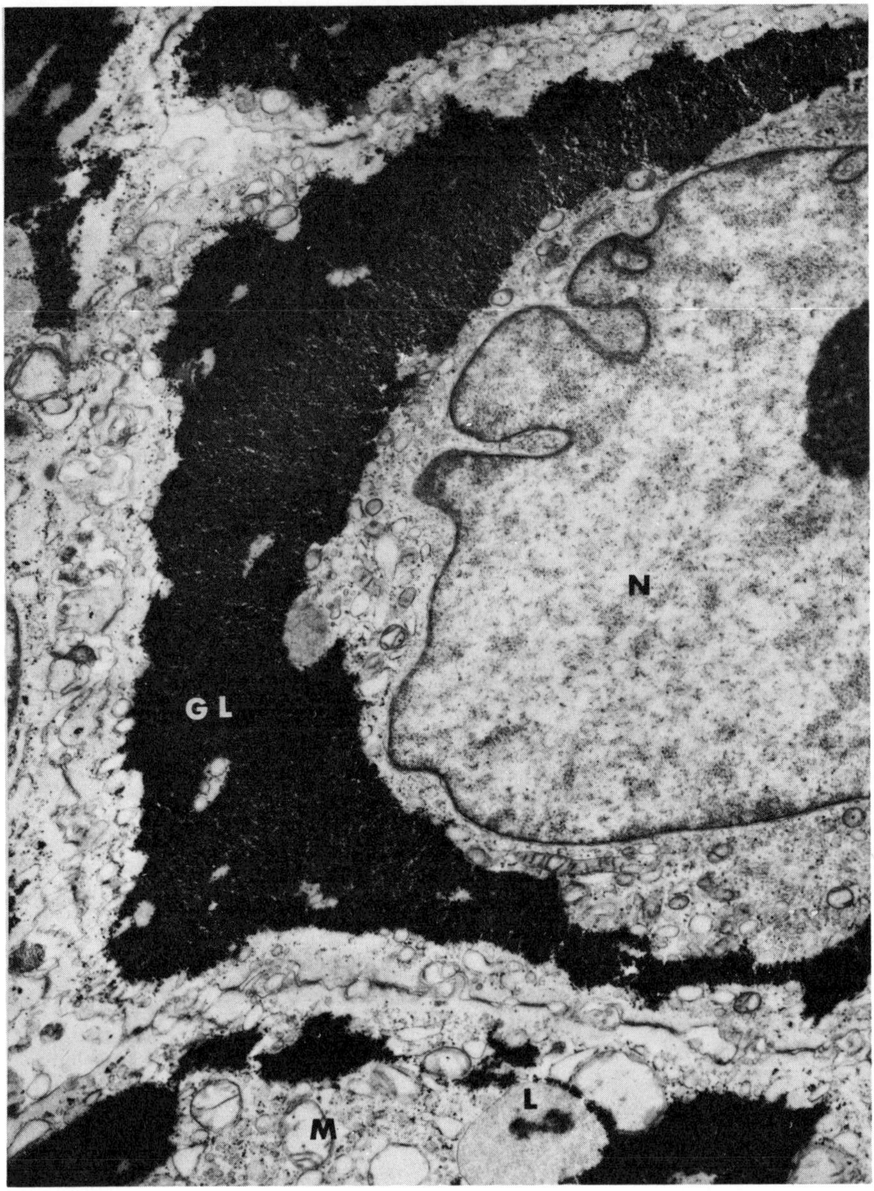

FIGURE 4. Electron micrograph of a BeWo trophoblast cell from a culture flask, showing heavy glycogen (GL) content; note the prominent desmosomes, Golgi apparatus, and lysosomes (L). N = nucleus; M = mitochondrion. (× 10,000)

blastic cell during adaptation to the *in vitro* environment. Stable levels of production of this glycoprotein have been documented, as shown in TABLE 1. Hormone production per cell per 24 hours has been previously reported as 1×10^{-5} IU (international unit) of HCG in the immature uterine weight bioassay of

TABLE 1
HUMAN CHORIONIC GONADOTROPIN PRODUCTION IN CELL CULTURE*

Cells per Flask	Cell Wet Weight (mg)	Sedimented Cell Quantity (cc)	HCG Production (IU/24 hours)
7.50×10^6	70	.07	70
7.50×10^6	71	.08	69
8.63×10^6	79	.08	81
7.89×10^6	72	.07	75
6.50×10^6	65	.06	62

*Average values from pooled 250-ml flasks: 10^8 cells/g/cc, producing 10^3 IU of HCG per 24 hours.

Delfs.[8] This approximate level has been attained in our study, and with larger volumes of cultures maintained in 250-ml flasks: Total cell counts have indicated one-hundred million cells with a wet weight of approximately 1 g/cc of sedimented cells, producing 1,000 IU of HCG in 24-hour incubations (0.1 mg of HCG).

The biological purity of the HCG produced by the trophoblast cell line was tested in the hypophysectomized immature female Sprague-Dawley rat. (Hypophysectomized animals were obtained from A. R. Schmidt, Madison, Wisconsin.) Hypophysectomy was carried out on the 19th or 20th day after birth, with assays performed 5 and 10 days following hypophysectomy in order to assure total elimination of any residual hormone from the animal's own pituitary gonadotrophins. The results of these assays, summarized in TABLE 2, show a complete lack of stimulation of ovarian or uterine response to 1,000 IU of HCG extracted from the medium in which the trophoblast cells were grown. Additional

TABLE 2
HUMAN CHORIONIC GONADOTROPIN BIOASSAYS IN HYPOPHYSECTOMIZED IMMATURE SPRAGUE-DAWLEY RATS

Hormone Administered*	Uterine Weight (mg)	Ovarian Weight (mg)	Ovarian Histology
1,000 IU HCG	16.5	11.2	Atrophic
	23.1	11.7	Atrophic
	18.0	12.3	Atrophic
	25.0	13.2	Atrophic
	23.0	12.1	Atrophic
Saline control	22.0	10.2	Atrophic
	26.0	8.2	Atrophic
1,000 IU HCG + 1.0 IU FSH	109.2	47.9	Stimulated
	79.0	34.0	Stimulated

*HCG = trophoblastic cellular human chorionic gonadotropic hormone; FSH supplied as Equinex®.

injections of up to 5,000 IU produced a similar lack of response. By contrast, when as little as 1.0 IU of follicle-stimulating hormone [FSH, supplied as Equinex® (Ayerst Laboratories, New York, N.Y.)] was added to the HCG injection, marked hyperstimulation of ovarian activity and uterine hypertrophy were observed. This assay paralleled the principle of the commonly used Steelman-Pohley bioassay.[9] From these results, it can be concluded that the trophoblastic cellular HCG produced has no intrinsic FSH property and is free from FSH contamination.

Human Placental Lactogen

Assays for the production of human placental lactogen (HPL) by the trophoblast cell line were determined on pooled medium incubated for 24 hours. The medium was chromatographed on a Sephadex G-100 column. Fractions were lyophylized and subsequently subjected to radioimmunoassay. Results indicated a low order of production of this polypeptide, with values of less than 2 μg/g of BeWo cells. The low values correlated well with the low order of production of HPL in patients with choriocarcinoma.

Steroid Biosynthesis

Steroid biosynthesis in the trophoblast cell line was determined by incubation of 25-cm^2 flask cultures with specific ^{3}H-labeled steroid precursors. Incubations were carried out for 24 hours in chemically defined medium at 37° C. Progesterone biosynthesis was demonstrated with 0.1 mg/ml of pregnenolone-7-^{3}H, containing 6 mc of radioactivity.

The reaction mixture was extracted with ether. The ether extract was partitioned between *n*-heptane and 80% methanol. The methanol fraction was subjected to alkali treatment to separate neutral and phenolic fractions. The neutral fraction was chromatographed on a Celite column. Radioactive progesterone was identified in the aliquot of radioactivity from the neutral fraction after authentic carrier progesterone and Δ^4-androstenedione were added (FIGURE 5). Superimposed radioactivity and optical density determinations yielded additional purification after pooling and rechromatographing.

These incubations established the presence of the crucial 3-β-ol dehydrogenase enzyme present in the normal placenta and responsible for the high level of conversion of pregnenolone to progesterone in normal pregnancy. Synthesis of estrone, estradiol, and estriol will be dealt with in subsequent reports.

Methotrexate Chemotherapy Studies

The availability of a pure source of malignant trophoblastic cells provided the opportunity for isolation of the enzyme inhibited by the antimetabolite

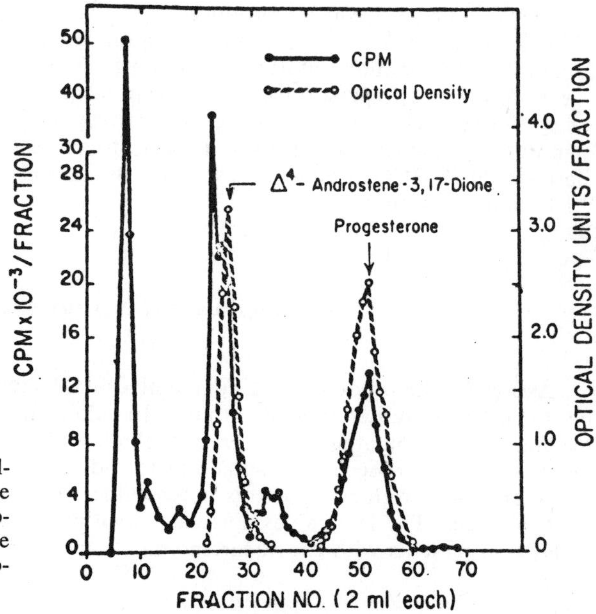

FIGURE 5. Partition column chromatography of the neutral fraction of the trophoblast cell line culture studied for progesterone biosynthesis.

methotrexate. Dihydrofolic reductase was isolated from flask cultures by means of Sephadex G-75 chromatography in tris-KC1 buffer, pH 7.0.

Methotrexate inhibits trophoblastic cell growth by inhibition of the production of THFA (tetrahydrofolic acid), thus preventing transfer of a methyl group from UdR (uracil deoxyribose) to TdR (thymidine deoxyribose synthetase). This inhibition was determined by measuring the decrease in radioactivity in the DNA fraction of cells incubated with 10^{-5}, 10^{-6}, 10^{-7}, and 10^{-8} molar concentrations (M) of methotrexate. The results (FIGURE 6) of incorporation of radioactivity into DNA, plotted as the percentage of inhibition, indicated a 100% inhibition by 10^{-5} M methotrexate; 90% inhibition by 10^{-6} M; 50% by 10^{-7} and 10^{-8} M; and no inhibition in controls.

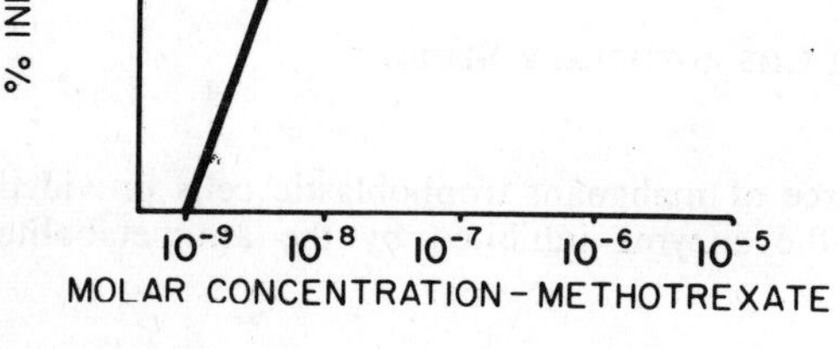

FIGURE 6. Incubation of the trophoblast cell line with ^{3}H-UdR at varying concentrations of methotrexate.

Chromosomes of the Trophoblast Cell Line

The trophoblast cell line has maintained a stable karyotype with a modal number of 78 to 86 chromosomes through over 150 passages. A single pair of long acrocentric chromosomes similar to those reported by Makino and his colleagues[10] has been observed.

Electrophysiology

Electrophoretic studies have shown that malignant cells possess a negative surface charge largely attributed to sialic acid-bearing mucopolysaccharides.[11] Lymphocytes have been shown to have a similar negative surface charge.[12] It has been postulated that malignant cells employ this negative surface charge to repel surface-negative lymphocytes, thus escaping normal immulogical mechanism and rejection phenomena.[13] The pregnant female fails to reject fetal trophoblast as an allograft, as is the case in choriocarcinoma, the invasive trophoblastic neoplasm following pregnancy.

Encouraged by the findings of a sialomucin cell coating similar to placental fibrinoid on the surface of malignant cells, together with the reports of an electrically charged surface on lymphocytes and malignant cells, we undertook an investigation to determine if the sialomucin coatings found on normal trophoblast and malignant cells imparted distinguishing characteristics to the cell surface which could be detected by direct single-cell penetration and bioelectrical recordings. Cells cultured on cover slips were studied in a specially designed chamber, which consisted of a bathing tray mounted on the stage of an inverted microscope, and contained a compartment for the cover slip culture immersed in culture medium maintained at 36° C, with pH and atmosphere controlled through CO_2 and air cannulas. Microelectrodes for cell penetration, accomplished with a micromanipulator, contained tip diameters of approximately 0.5 μ and were filled with 2 M KCl. Electrical recordings were obtained through a high-input impedance bioelectrical amplifier and stored on tape.

Cells from the malignant BeWo choriocarcinoma line were examined first. Cell penetration revealed a prominent transmembrane potential of 35–50 mv, the lower value at pH 7 and the higher value at pH 8.0. A notable positive prepotential preceded the typical negative transmembrane potential (FIGURE 7). This prepotential was associated with a surface phenomena encountered before membrane impalement and suggests the presence of a cell-surface coating inscribing a distinct ionic layer. The positive prepotential was accentuated at high pH and dropped to 2 mμ at pH 7.0–7.3. A proposed thesis for the positive-prepotential finding by direct impalement instead of the negative surface charge found in electrophoresis is diagrammed in FIGURE 8. The extracellular media is held at zero reference by a silver chloride indifferent electrode. At position 1, the electrode tip is at zero potential, and no deflection is produced. At position 2, the electrode tip is within the mucopolysaccharide coating, which is structured so that the electronegative sialic acid[14] moiety is a *terminal* group. This provides the negatively charged terminal group and external media with a

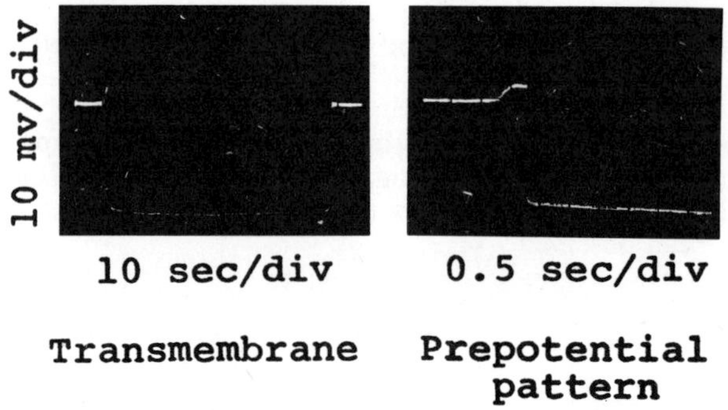

FIGURE 7. Single-cell penetration with a microelectrode, showing the positive prepotential and sharp negative transmembrane potential found in all malignant cells studied.

continuum referenced toward the indifferent electrode with the selective electrode tip positioned near the positive outer surface of the cell membrane proper. Thus, a positive deflection develops at position 2. At position 3, the electrode tip experiences a highly negative intracellular environment and gives the classical transmembrane depolarization.

Similar recordings were made and examined from up to 100 cells from malignant human rat tumors in culture; from the malignant and normal human trophoblast, both in culture and, in one case, trophoblastic cells directly from a patient on the 28th day of pregnancy when the specimen was obtained from the cervical canal during a spontaneous abortion (sections from the trophoblast of this specimen were examined and found to be histologically normal); from human lymphocytes in culture; and from cultures of normal human embryonic heart, kidney, and lung tissues. The results (TABLE 3) show that all trophoblastic cells and lymphocytic cells displayed a normal transmembrane potential and a positive prepotential, whereas normal cells from heart and kidney generally did not show the prepotential. Human embroyonic lung cells occasionally showed a

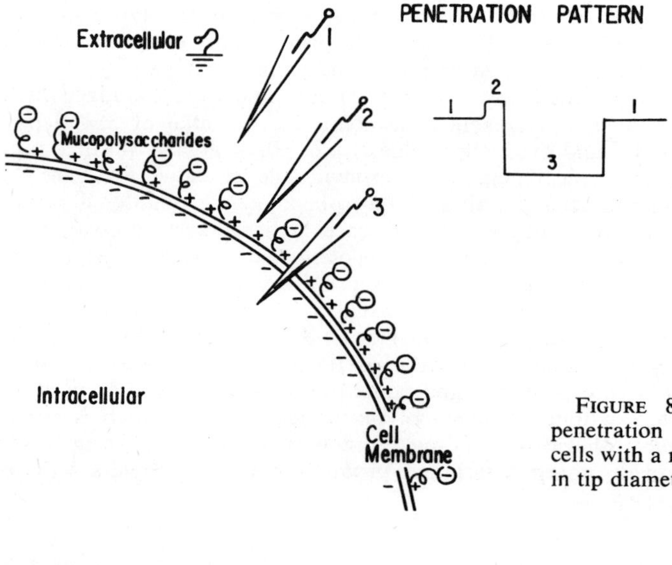

FIGURE 8. Diagram of the penetration pattern of single cells with a microelectrode 0.5 μ in tip diameter.

positive prepotential; however, these were generally in cells late in the mitotic process and may reflect increased sialic acid levels during the mitotic process.[15]

These studies have shown the presence of a similar charged surface on malignant cells, trophoblast cells, and lymphocytes. This charge was generally not present on normal cells. The charge seems to correlate with the previously reported presence of sialomucin[16] identified on the surface of malignant and

TABLE 3

COMPARATIVE CELL PENETRATIONS

Cell	Prepotential (mv)	Transmembrane Potential (mv)
BeWo trophoblast cell (choriocarcinoma)	+5–+8	−35
Trophoblast cell from a 28-day pregnancy (spontaneous abortion)	+4	− 5
HEp-2 (laryngial cancer)	+5	−30
Sarcoma-256	+2–+4	−20
Normal human lymphocyte	+4–+8	−12
Normal human embryonic heart	—	−35
Normal human embryonic kidney	—	−20
WI-38 (normal human lung)	±	−25

trophoblast cells. The role of this sialomucin in producing the charged surfaces found in this study and its role in immunological protection in gestation and cancer will require further biochemical investigation.

SUMMARY

Studies of endocrine metabolism in trophoblastic tumor cells in cell culture have been reported. Biosynthesis of glycoprotein and steroid hormones have shown that each of the normal pathways thus far tested is present in these cells in culture. Further studies are necessary to identify any possible deviation from the normal pathways. Preliminary studies of ultrastructure, chemotherapy, immunological mechanisms, and electrophysiological properties have been reported.

ACKNOWLEDGMENTS

The authors wish to thank Dr. M. H. Kauffman, Department of Surgery, Marquette School of Medicine, for supplying lymphocytes for culture; Dr. M. Rytel, Department of Medicine (Infectious Diseases), Marquette School of Medicine, for supplying L-cells; and Mr. D. Nelson, State Laboratory of Hygiene, Virology Section, Madison, Wisconsin, for WI-38 and HEp-2 cells. We deeply appreciate the technical assistance of Miss A. Ruckert, Mr. J. Kurtz, Mrs. J. Martin and Mr. Richard Falsetti.

REFERENCES

1. HERTIG, A. 1966. *In* Williams Obstetrics. N. J. Eastman & E. M. Hellman, Eds. 13th edit.: 120. Appleton-Century-Crofts, Inc. New York, N.Y.
2. HRESHCHYSHYN, M. M., C. HACKER & N. R. ROSE. 1968. Quantitation of urinary chorionic gonadotropins by hemagglutination inhibition technique. Amer. J. Obstet. Gynec. **101**: 269–271.
3. SPELLACY, W. N., K. L. CARLSON & S. A. BIRK. 1966. Dynamics of human placental lactogen. Amer. J. Obstet. Gynec. **96**: 1164–1173.
4. HASEGAWA, T., G. NOZUE, S. SHINTANI & I. TAKAHARA. 1967. Trophoblastic neoplasias as they are in Japan (3rd Report). Fifth World Congr. Gynec. Obstet.: 411. Appleton-Century-Crofts, Inc. New York, N.Y.
5. HERTZ, R. 1959. Choriocarcinoma of women maintained in serial passage in hamster and rat. Proc. Soc. Exp. Biol. Med. **102**: 77–80.
6. PATTILLO, R. A. & G. O. GEY. 1968. The establishment of a cell line of human hormone-synthesizing trophoblastic cells *in vitro*. Cancer Res. **28**: 1231–1236.
7. VILLEE, C. A., H. VAN LEUSDEN & L. ZELEWSKI. 1965. The regulation of the biosynthesis of sterols and steroids in the placenta. Advances Enzyme Reg. **4**: 165.
8. DELFS, E. 1959. Chorionic gonadotrophin determinations in patients with hydatidiform mole and choriocarcinoma. Ann. N. Y. Acad. Sci. **80**(1): 125–139.
9. STEELMAN, S. L. & F. M. POHLEY. 1953. Assay of the follicle stimulating hormone based on the augmentation with human chorionic gonadotrophin. Endocrinology **53**: 604–616.
10. MAKINO, S., M. S. SASAKI & T. FUKUSCHIMA. 1965. Cytological studies of tumors. XLI. Chromosomal instability in human chorionic lesions. Okajima. Folia Anat. Jap. **40**: 439–465.
11. FORRESTER, J. A., E. J. AMBROSE & I. MCPHERSON. 1962. Nature **196**: 1068.
12. ROBINAUX, R. & S. BOGIN. 1951. Sang **22**: 241.
13. CURRIE, G. A. & K. D. BAGSHAWE. 1967. The masking of antigens on trophoblast and cancer cells. Lancet **i**: 708–710.
14. GOTTSCHALK, A. 1960. Relation between composition, structure, shape and function of a salivary muco-protein. Nature **186**: 949–951.
15. CARUBELLI, R. & M. J. GRIFFIN. 1967. Sialic acid in HeLa cells: Effect of hydrocortisone. Science **157**: 693–694.
16. GASIC, G. & T. BEYDAK. 1961. Biological Interractions in Normal and Neoplastic Growth. M. J. Brennan & W. L. Simpson, Eds.: 709. Little, Brown & Co. Boston, Mass.

THE PATHOLOGY OF CHORIOCARCINOMA

William B. Ober,* M.D., John H. Edgcomb,† M.D.
and Edward B. Price, Jr.,‡ M.D.

Pathological Anatomy Branch, National Cancer Institute
National Institutes of Health, Bethesda, Md.

INTRODUCTION

Eleven years ago The New York Academy of Sciences published a monograph entitled "Trophoblast and its Tumors."[1] It was only 2 or 3 years prior to this publication that an era of chemotherapy in the management of choriocarcinoma had begun. Since then, there has been a dramatic decrease in mortality from this malignant tumor, which was formerly almost invariably fatal. Now, under optimal conditions, long-term survival rates on the order of 90% have been obtained in several clinics.

The first extensive publication in English on choriocarcinoma was in 1903 by the late John H. Teacher;[2] in 1950 a review of the subject was written by Park and Lees.[3] Three recent monographs have summarized current knowledge about the placenta, human trophoblast, and choriocarcinoma: Benirschke's and Driscoll's "The Pathology of the Human Placenta,"[4] Hertig's "Human Trophoblast,"[5] and Bagshawe's "Choriocarcinoma."[6] Reference to these texts makes a historical review of the subject redundant. This paper is limited to a study of pathological material accessioned to the files of the Pathological Anatomy Branch of the National Cancer Institute, National Institutes of Health (NIH), between 1953 and 1963 from 100 women with choriocarcinoma. These women represent a series of admisisons to hospital; several received little or no treatment, but no woman with choriocarcinoma was dropped from the series.

At this point it is proper to point out an important difference between the role of the clinician and the role of the morbid anatomist with respect to a patient with choriocarcinoma or some other trophoblastic disease. The clinician is confronted with a patient suffering from a disease that is potentially malignant, and his duty is to devise a rational basis for therapy. In practice, this involves study of the patient's history and physical and roentgenographic findings, determination of the titer of human chorionic gonadotropin (HCG), and consideration of whatever histopathological evidence may be available. The pathologist, confronted by a specimen of tissue, must assign to it some meaningful anatomical classification. In practice, even before the days of chemotherapy, accurate anatomical diagnosis of the disease in the patient could not always be made from competent examination of biopsies and surgical specimens, and was thus sometimes deferred until autopsy. The difficulty in predicting the subsequent behavior

*Present address: Attending Pathologist, Beth Israel Hospital, and Associate Professor of Pathology, The Mount Sinai School of Medicine, New York, N.Y.

†Present address: Pathologist, Gorgas Memorial Laboratory, Balboa Heights, Canal Zone.

‡Present address: Pathologist, Armed Forces Institute of Pathology, Washington, D.C.

of trophoblastic lesions by the examination of uterine curettings is well known to pathologists.

Under these circumstances, Hertz and his colleagues[7] have developed the clinical concept of *persistent trophoblastic disease,* a term that includes several types of potentially malignant trophoblastic lesions not classifiable as choriocarcinoma but requiring chemotherapy. For the best results, the clincian treating a patient with chemotherapeutic agents must diagnose the presence of abnormal trophoblast as quickly as he can, and he must administer these agents as soon as possible in sufficient amounts to destroy the trophoblast completely. Delays are regularly associated with failure. These inexorable requirements of successful chemotherapy have changed the relationship of clinician and pathologist in the diagnosis and management of choriocarcinoma and related diseases. Sensitive and accurate endocrinological and immunological assays of chorionic gonadotropins may demonstrate the presence of abnormal trophoblast in a patient when anatomical diagnosis is difficult or impossible. Chorionic gonadotropin assays are much more valuable and much more sensitive than is any histopathological procedure in assessing the effectiveness of chemotherapy during treatment, and in following treated patients to be sure that they remain free of recurrent disease. The consensus of clinical experience is that the patient's best interests are served by carefully managed chemotherapy even in the absence of anatomical support for the diagnosis of a malignant trophoblastic neoplasm. Persistent trophoblastic disease includes such definable entities as (*1*) invasive hydatidiform mole (chorioadenoma destruens), (*2*) hydatidiform mole with persistently elevated HCG titer, (*3*) hydatidiform mole with pulmonary deportation demonstrated roetgenographically, (*4*) hydatidiform mole complicated by a trophoblast-containing vaginal nodule, and (*5*) retained hydatidiform mole, as well as other entities less well-defined. Park[8] has invented the term *clinical choriomatosis* to include these various entities, and this term has a practical value similar to that of Hertz and co-workers.[7]

The material we have studied during this period of decreased mortality would be rare under any conditions; with the present improvements in diagnosis and therapy, it should cease to exist from now on. Useful descriptions of the pathology of choriocarcinoma are those by Novak and Seah,[9] who in 1954 reported 74 cases from the files of the Mathieu Chorionepithelioma Registry (their valuable contribution to the literature is somewhat limited by the nature of the pathological material contributed to the Registry from many clinical sources); by Hou and Pang,[10] who in 1956 reported their observations on 28 autopsied cases of choriocarcinoma (detailed clinical information was not available to them); and by Smalbraak,[11] who in 1957 presented clinical and pathological data about 17 patients diagnosed as having choriocarcinoma, all of whom were observed at one clinic during the period 1927–1952.

The present report presents experience of 100 consecutive choriocarcinomas, all in women referred to a single clinic for treatment. The cases have been selected from a larger group in which definitive diagnosis of choriocarcinoma by pathological criteria could not be made, but most of whom were treated for persistent trophoblastic disease. These cases have been divided into five groups (TABLE 1). Most patients in these groups were treated with methotrexate and other chemotherapeutic agents by Li and his colleagues[12] and by Hertz and his associates,[7,13] who supplied detailed clinical histories, methods of treatment, and notes on the patients' subsequent clinical courses. In this report, only the most pertinent clinical and endocrinological data will be repeated. In all patients except those in Group V, the diagnosis of choriocarcinoma has been histologically verified; the four cases included in this group are presented to demonstrate

TABLE 1

CLASSIFICATION OF CHORIOCARCINOMA AT THE NATIONAL CANCER INSTITUTE: 1952–1962

Group	Classification	Case Nos.	No. of Cases
I	Gestational choriocarcinoma, fatal, autopsied	1–44	44
II	Gestational choriocarcinoma, fatal, not autopsied	45–50	6
III	Nongestational choriocarcinoma, fatal, autopsied	51–54	4
IV	Gestational choriocarcinoma, nonfatal, histologically verified	55–96	42
V	Probable gestational choriocarcinoma, nonfatal	97–100	4
			100

the limitations of histopathological diagnosis even in the face of the strongest presumption.

Of the 96 cases of gestational choriocarcinoma, 87 are considered to be chemotherapeutically treated cases, i.e., to have received at least one full course of methotrexate, and nine are considered to be untreated cases managed by procedures other than chemotherapy. Some of these nine cases were treated before the development of chemotherapy, and others, admitted moribund, died before a full course could be given. Three of the four women with nongestational choriocarcinoma were treated with chemotherapeutic agents. Since nongestational choriocarcinoma is in many respects different from gestational choriocarcinoma, these will be considered separately.

A prerequisite for admission to the clinical services of the National Cancer Institute for treatment of choriocarcinoma or persistent trophoblastic disease is the presentation of convincing evidence of correct diagnosis by the referring physician. Consequently, at least one histopathological section from each patient was available for study. The sections were received from many contributing laboratories and varied in quantity, quality, and relevance. In the vast majority of cases, the contributed sections were sufficient for diagnosis; in only a few instances did review of contributed sections leave serious questions unanswered. In most of these instances, however, tissue obtained subsequently was diagnostic.

Surgical and autopsy material was fixed in neutral formalin and stained routinely with hematoxylin and eosin. Selected sections were stained by Masson's trichrome technique, the Verhoeff-van Gieson method for elastic tissue and collagen, the Hotchkiss-McManus periodic acid-leukofuchsin method, Mallory's phosphotungstic acid hematoxylin method, Glenner's aldehyde-fuchsin method (for the pituitary gland), and the Gaulin-Gagarin method (for pancreatic islets).

The method for determining quantitative urinary chorionic gonadotropin values is that of Klinefelter and co-workers,[14] using Albert's kaolin-acetone method of extraction. The test animal is the immature female mouse, and the end point is uterine weight. Values are expressed in mouse units per 24 hours; 1 mouse unit is equivalent to 0.1 international unit (IU).

OBSERVATIONS

Age, Race, Gravidity, and Parity

The 100 patients ranged between 9 and 51 years of age, with a mean age of 28.9 years. The mean age at onset of 44 fatal, autopsied cases was 31.6 years;

the mean age at onset of 42 nonfatal cases was 26.5 years. In those patients in whom choriocarcinoma followed term delivery, the mean age at onset in 18 fatal cases was 30.3 years, whereas in 19 nonfatal cases it was 24.3 years. Ninety patients were white; ten were black.

In the 96 patients with gestational choriocarcinoma, there were 305 known conceptions with 208 live-born, apparently healthy children (68%). These 96 patients had had 54 nonmolar abortions, at least one of which had been procured extralegally, and 38 hydatidiform moles. Three patients had had two spontaneous nonmolar abortions, and one had had three. No patient had had more than one hydatidiform mole, but two patients who had had a previous hydatidiform mole later developed choriocarcinoma of the uterus after a term delivery. Three of the four patients with nongestational choriocarcinoma were nulligravidae; one of these was 9 and another 16 years old; the third had never menstruated. Of the 96 patients with gestational choriocarcinoma, 24 were primigravidae (25%), and 22 had had five or more pregnancies (23%). No significant difference was found when comparing the number of pregnancies following hydatidiform mole with the number of pregnancies following term delivery or nonmolar abortion.

Type of Antecedent Pregnancy

The nature of the gestation preceding the development of choriocarcinoma in 96 patients with gestational choriocarcinoma is summarized in TABLE 2. It is noteworthy that more patients in this series developed choriocarcinoma following term delivery (40) than after a hydatidiform mole (34). An example of choriocarcinoma developing after hysterectomy for chorioadenoma destruens will be described in detail (case 31).

TABLE 2

TYPE OF ANTECEDENT GESTATION IN GESTATIONAL CHORIOCARCINOMA

Type of Gestation	Group				Total	Total Fatal	Total Nonfatal
	I	II	IV	V			
Term delivery	18	1	19	2	40	19	21
Hydatidiform mole	17	3	13	1	34	20	14
Abortion	7	2	10	0	19	9	10
Uncertain	2	0	0	1	3	2	1
Total	44	6	42	4	96	50	46

In some patients, it was not possible to be certain about the nature of the gestation from which the choriocarcinoma arose. Some bizarre anamnestic situations were encountered. For example, a 51-year-old woman (case 32), the oldest patient in the series, had been curetted of a hydatidiform mole 4 years previously, and total amenorrhea followed. After this lapse of 4 years, vaginal bleeding led to curettage, and tissue diagnostic of choriocarcinoma was removed. The possibility that the choriocarcinoma developed following a subclinical abortion cannot be excluded. Another patient, a 39-year-old gravida 2, para 2 (case 48), developed vaginal bleeding, and curettage revealed choriocarcinoma. Her younger child was 10 years old, and she denied having had sexual relations for the past 4 or 5 years. That she could have had regular menses and a uterine choriocarcinoma for 10 years seems unlikely. Cases 43 and 44 are other examples of exceptional clinical histories. There are data in this and other large series of cases of choriocarcinoma which cannot be fitted into rigid categories or fixed sequences, and we have reservations about similar data in other series in which every case is confidently assigned to a specific antecedent gestation.

Fetal Sex in Cases of Choriocarcinoma following Term Delivery

Information about the sex of the fetus was recorded in 33 of 37 patients who developed choriocarcinoma following term delivery. There were 18 female and 15 male infants. In 18 fatal cases, there were ten female and eight male infants; in 19 nonfatal cases, there were eight female and seven male infants; sex was not recorded in four cases. This observation is in agreement with that of Schoen and co-workers[15] that there is no sex preference in pregnancies eventuating in choriocarcinoma. We infer from these data that the genetic sex of the trophoblast is not related to its response to chemotherapy. This inference is consistent with Park's observation[16] that there is no demonstrable difference in mortality in patients whose tumors were classed male or female according to the nuclear sex-chromatin (22 hydatidiform moles and 26 choriocarcinomas); those with low sex-chromatin counts (male) were as lethal as those with high sex-chromatin counts (female).

Chronological Sequences in Choriocarcinoma

It is rarely possible to assign a specific date or a specific anatomical site to the beginning of a choriocarcinoma. Clemmer and Hansmann[17] have shown that choriocarcinoma may arise from trophoblastic cells that have migrated from the site of placentation to loci deep in the myometrium. Driscoll[18] has described a focus of choriocarcinomatous tissue in a term placenta; neither mother nor child showed evidence of disease. Brewer and Gerbie[19] have reported a similar case in which choriocarcinoma was seen in a term placenta. Choriocarcinoma rarely presents as a recognizable tumor coincident with pregnancy, but MacRae[20] has reported such a case, and there are two case reports in which both mother and child were affected.[21,22] The usual sequence of events is the delivery of products of conception, be they abortal, molar, or normal, followed by clinical presentation of the neoplasm. In patients in whom there is no definable antecedent gestation, clinical suspicion may be slow to develop, and diagnosis may be delayed. If the choriocarcinoma arises from the immediately antecedent pregnancy, a maximum time limit can be set. For example, a patient in whom gestational choriocarcinoma is diagnosed from curettings 1 month postpartum cannot have harbored neoplastic trophoblast for longer than 10 months, and it is probable that the neoplastic change occurred after the pregnancy was well established. The chronological limit is different from most other neoplasms, which may have been present and growing slowly for several years before becoming clinically manifest. In choriocarcinoma, certain dates can be established, namely, the date of delivery, the date a mole was passed, or the date of onset of bleeding in a nonmolar abortion. Based on such available data, it is possible to detect differences with respect to time in the behavior of choriocarcinoma developing after term delivery as opposed to choriocarcinoma following a hydatidiform mole. (TABLE 3).

TABLE 3

CHRONOLOGY OF CHORIOCARCINOMA IN RELATION TO THE TYPE OF ANTECEDENT GESTATION

Type of Antecedent Gestation	No. of Cases		Mean Interval between Gestation and Diagnosis (months)	Mean Interval between Gestation and Death (months)
	Total	Fatal		
Term pregnacy	24	9	2	11*
Hydatidiform mole	23	12†	9	28‡
Abortion	12	6	5	11

*Only one case survived longer than 12 months.

†Excluding one case of choriocarcinoma developing from a chorioadenoma destruens (invasive hydatidiform mole).

‡Only two cases survived less than 12 months.

Of 37 patients who developed choriocarcinoma following term delivery, the major presenting symptom was abnormal vaginal bleeding, either continuous or discontinuous, in 28 instances. In 14 patients, bleeding was continuous from the time of delivery; in the other 14, it presented as delayed postpartum bleeding at an interval of 2 to 8 weeks after delivery. Histopathological diagnosis of choriocarcinoma was established in 21 of these patients at intervals ranging from 4 to 10 weeks postpartum. Certain exceptional cases may be mentioned: In one instance, vaginal bleeding developed at 8 weeks postpartum, and severe lumbar pain at 12 weeks; a chest x-ray film showed multiple bilateral nodular densities, and the urinary HCG was elevated. The correct clinical diagnosis of choriocarcinoma was made but not verified until autopsy 10 months postpartum. In another patient, vaginal bleeding at 8 weeks was treated by cervical cauterization; at 12 weeks there was recurrence of vaginal bleeding concomitant with projectile vomiting and other signs of an expanding intracranial mass. The histopathological diagnosis of choriocarcinoma was established at emergency craniotomy. In a third patient, tubal ligation was performed following a third cesarean section for pelvic disproportion. After 15 months of somewhat irregular menses, vaginal spotting occurred, followed a few days later by massive hemoptysis; the histological diagnosis of choriocarcinoma was made following pulmonary lobectomy for what was thought to be a single metastatic nodule. In a fourth patient, choriocarcinoma was diagnosed 4 months postpartum on a hysterectomy specimen after a curettage at 6 weeks for delayed postpartum bleeding showed only secretory endometrium. In a fifth patient, biopsy of a fungating ischiorectal mass 9 weeks postpartum yielded a diagnosis of choriocarcinoma after two prior curettages for postpartum hemorrhages at 3 and 5 weeks had not proved diagnostic.

But in most patients with choriocarcinoma following term delivery, a histological diagnosis is made by examining uterine curettings 1 to 3 months after delivery. The curettage has usually been performed to determine the cause of abnormal postpartum bleeding. Of 18 fatal cases of choriocarcinoma developing postpartum, survival time ranged from 2 to 18 months; mean survival time was 7 months. Only one fatality survived longer than 12 months from the initiation of treatment.

Patients who developed choriocarcinoma following a hydatidiform mole had more varied clinical courses and longer spans of disease. In 17 fatal cases of postmolar choriocarcinoma, survival time ranged from 5 to 32 months, with a mean survival time of 11 months after the diagnosis of choriocarcinoma. Only two patients survived for less than ayear from the time of passage or evacuation of the mole.

In 30 patients with postmolar choriocarcinoma, the average interval between passage of the mole and definitive diagnosis of choriocarcinoma was 13 months (with range of 1 to 48 months). In five cases, clinical diagnoses of choriocarcinoma were verified only at autopsy. Histological diagnosis was established by uterine curettings in ten patients, biopsy of a vaginal nodule in one, pulmonary lobectomy in five, and hysterectomy in seven. Two hysterectomies were performed because of uncontrollable bleeding at the time of evacuation of the mole. In this group, eight hysterectomies were performed for persistent vaginal bleeding accompanied by elevated HCG titers after one or more (up to four) prior curettages had failed to yield material suitable for diagnosis.

Evaluation of curettings after evacuation of a mole is a pathological problem quite different from the evaluation of postpartum curettings. The presence of retained chorionic villi almost invariably excludes a diagnosis of choriocarcinoma. Infiltration of superficial myometrium by exuberant trophoblast may mimic the morphology of a non-neoplastic postmolar placental site reaction (so-called syncytial endometritis) so closely that diagnosis of the material received may not be possible. Commitment to a diagnosis of choriocarcinoma on the basis of insufficient material is a constant danger. As a practical matter, it is much easier to make a histopathological diagnosis of postpartum choriocarcinoma than of postmolar choriocarcinoma. However, delay in diagnosis does not seem to be the principal factor in the relatively longer survival of patients with postmolar choriocarcinoma. Postmolar choriocarcinomas seem to differ in their biological behavior from postpartum choriocarcinomas, but it is not known what accounts for the difference.

Choriocarcinoma developing after a nonmolar abortion more closely resembles the behavior of a postpartum choriocarcinoma than a postmolar one. In 12 patients with postabortal choriocarcinoma, the prominent symptom was continuous, intermittent, or delayed vaginal bleeding. Diagnosis was established by curettage in nine patients at intervals ranging from 2 to 13 months after the date of abortion; the mean interval was 5 months. In two patients, diagnosis was established by hysterectomy, previous curettage having failed to yield a diagnosis, and in one patient by biopsy of a vaginal nodule. In seven fatal cases of postabortal choriocarcinoma, the mean survival was 11 months, with a range of 9 to 15 months. These observations do not support the speculation that there is some relationship between the length of survival and the age of the trophoblast at the time neoplastic transformation occurs.

Clinical manifestations and chronological sequences in the four patients with nongestational choriocarcinoma are quite different, and are presented in the epitomes of these cases (Group III, cases 51–54).

Clinical Manifestations and Methods of Diagnosis

In this series, there are 48 examples of histologically verified choriocarcinoma which proved fatal; 44 of these were autopsied, and four were not. The histopathological diagnosis of choriocarcinoma was established by microscopical examination of uterine curettings in 15 patients; and two other patients, choriocarcinoma was present in the uterus and in curettings when hysterectomies and curettages were done simultaneously. In six patients, correct clinical diagnoses were confirmed at autopsy but could not be made before that. Uterine curettage failed to provide diagnostic tissue in six patients (five postmolar, one antecedent gestation unclassified) despite strong presumptive grounds for the clinical diagnosis; histopathological diagnoses were made in these patients on hysterectomy specimens. Tissue diagnosis was established by craniotomy in two patients, biopsy of a vaginal nodule in four, pulmonary lobectomy or lung biopsy in five, resection of a loop of small bowel in four, and nephrectomy in one.

In the six patients in whom a tissue diagnosis was not established until autopsy, the uterus was free of tumor. Curettages in three of them had shown only decidua or secretory endometrium. The clinical diagnosis of choriocarcinoma was confirmed at autopsy by finding metastatic deposits in various organs, but there was no evidence in the uteri that a choriocarcinoma had been there as a primary focus and had then undergone regression.

In the 48 histologically verified fatal cases, a chest x-ray film was positive in 43 patients (89%) for metastatic tumor nodules, bilateral in most instances. Clinical signs and symptoms of intracranial metastases were present in 32 of 50 fatal cases (64%), and in 21 of these the intracarnial metastases were considered to be the principal cause of death. Massive gastrointestinal hemorrhage from ulcerated metastases was a clinical problem in seven patients and a cause of death in three. Massive intraperitoneal hemorrhage caused death in five patients, by rupture of hepatic metastases in four and by by rupture of a primary uterine tumor that had perforated the uterine wall in one. Respiratory failure caused by pulmonary metastases was prominent in the terminal clinical state of five patients, two of which also had large intracerebral metastases. One patient died with cor pulmonale and right-sided cardiac failure from multiple obstructive intravascular metastases.

In ten patients, drug toxicity played an important role in the antemortem clinical picture, one of leukopenia and bacteremia due to gram-negative bacilli. Toxicity of some degree is regularly associated with the chemotherapy employed, and is, in most cases, reversible on cessation of treatment. It should be emphasized that these deaths occurred during a period of early experience with chemotherapy in patients with "drug-resistant" disease, almost all of whom had widely disseminated metastases. An element of oversimplification is implicit in assigning causes of death in a group of patients, treated or untreated, with widely disseminated choriocarcinoma; each patient died from a multiplicity of factors acting in concert.

In the 42 histologically verified nonfatal cases, the tissue diagnosis was established on uterine curettings in 25 (three of these with concomitant positive hysterectomy specimens). In nine patients, the diagnosis of choriocarcinoma was made on hysterectomy specimens; in five of these, previous curettages had not been diagnostic. In one patient, the diagnosis was established by simultaneous curettage and biopsy of a vaginal nodule; in four patients, the diagnosis was made on biopsy of a vaginal nodule (and confirmed at subsequent hysterectomy). In one patient, the diagnosis was established by pulmonary lobectomy for a coin lesion discovered 9 years after passage of a hydatidiform mole, and in another by excision of a pulmonary coin lesion 8 months after a mole. In one patient who developed delayed postpartum bleeding at 3.5 weeks, two curettages yielded only secretory endometrium; the diagnosis was established by biopsy of a fungating ischiorectal mass 8 weeks postpartum. Pretreatment chest x-ray films were interpreted as positive for metastatic disease in 31 of the 42 surviving patients (74%), equivocal in one patient, and negative in ten.

Mortality

In series of cases of choriocarcinoma collected before the introduction of effective chemotherapy, mortality has ranged from 80 to 100%. Spontaneous regression is rare; Everson and Cole's comprehensive monograph[23] lists only 17 documented cases in women. A number of cases in which trophoblastic disease not diagnosed as choriocarcinoma has persisted for a time and then regressed have been described,[24] but these cases are not acceptable as true choriocarcinoma with spontaneous regression. A summary of recent reported series (TABLE 4) in the years preceding chemotherapy suggests the mortality to be on the order of 81%. Clearly, some patients do survive after hysterectomy alone, and there are numerous isolated reports of regression or survival following a variety of therapeutic measures given in desperation or for want of something better: nitrogen mustard therapy combined with radiotherapy, pituitary ablation with yttrium-90, hormone therapy, treatment with serum from pregnant women, etc.

TABLE 4
RESULTS OF TREATMENT OF CHORIOCARCINOMA BEFORE THE DAYS OF CHEMOTHERAPY

Author	No. of Cases	Survivors
Novak	74	13
Iverson	57	11
Brews	24	8
Smalbraak	17	7
Brewer	147	21
Douglas	24	7
Siegler	11	5
Dilworth	11	0
King	15	3
Soma	22	5
Mitani	16	2
Hunter	18	2
Total	436	84 (19%)

In the present series of 96 cases of gestational choriocarcinoma including ten untreated cases, the overall mortality was 52% (TABLE 5). Of the 80 histologically verified, treated patients with gestational choriocarcinomas, 40 patients were living, well, and free from endocrine or roentgenographic evidence of choriocarcinoma for 5 years or more after the cessation of therapy—a survival rate of 50%. This statistic is already out of date; survival following treatment with methotrexate, actinomycin-D, and chlorambucil (alone and in various combinations) is on the order of 90%. Many patients in this series received treatment when they had far advanced and widely disseminated disease. The more favorable results depend on their earlier application of chemotherapy. This has become a reality as physicians become aware that chemotherapy is more often successful than not and with the development of treatment centers staffed by experienced personnel and supported by appropriate laboratory facilities.

Bagshawe and Wilde[25] have reported that of 37 patients with pelvic choriocarcinoma treated with methotrexate and 6-mercaptopurine, 31 (84%) had a

TABLE 5

MORTALITY OF GESTATIONAL CHORIOCARCINOMA*

	Dead	Surviving	Mortality Rate (%)
Total cases (96)	50	46	52
Histologically verified cases only (90)	48	42	53
Treated cases (80)	40	40	50
Untreated cases (10)	8	2	80

*Excluding the four cases of nongestational choriocarcinoma.

complete remission. The present report includes four fatal cases of nongestational choriocarcinoma in complex ovarian neoplasms. Wider and co-workers[26] cite three similar patients with sustained remissions lasting 14 months to 4.5 years after treatment with methotrexate, actinomycin-D, and chlorambucil. (Case 4 in their series, dying 13 months after operation, is identical with case 53 in this series.)

Two cases in this series support the observation that a patient with choriocinoma occasionally is cured by hysterectomy. One patient (case 59) was diagnosed as having choriocarcinoma 8 weeks after term delivery on the basis of uterine curettings. Hysterectomy and bilateral salpingo-oophorectomy were promptly performed, and abundant residual choriocarcinoma was found to be invading the uterus some distance away from the normally involuting placental site. Four months later, the HCG titer was 200–300 mouse units, and the chest x-ray film was clear. No chemotherapy was given, and the patient has remained well for more than 10 years. Another patient (case 79) underwent hysterectomy for choriocarcinoma 5 months after a hydatidiform mole. Two months later, the HCG titer was 200–500 mouse units, and the chest x-ray film was clear. No treatment was given, and she too has been free from evidence of disease, for nearly 7 years.

MORBID ANATOMY OF CHORIOCARCINOMA

The 96 cases of gestational choriocarcinoma can be subdivided into those in which the primary tumor was examined at autopsy, at hysterectomy, by curetting, or not at all. All four cases of nongestational choriocarcinoma arose in the ovary as parts of complex neoplasms. Of the 100 patients, 31 (including the four nongestational cases) did not have diagnostic curettages. In the 69 patients who did, the tissue was positive for choriocarcinoma in 49 (71%). Of the 20 patients in whom curettage did not yield diagnostic tissue, the uterus contained choriocarcinoma in eight cases, and healed or necrotic lesions were found in four; therefore, in 12 (60%) of those patients with negative curettings, there was evidence of present or past uterine choriocarcinoma.

In 27 patients, the initial histopathological diagnosis of choriocarcinoma was established by examination of tissue other than curettings or the uterus. In the four patients with nongestational choriocarcinoma, the diagnosis was established by examination of the ovarian tumor. In the other 23 cases, diagnosis was established by examination of vaginal nodule (nine cases), lung biopsy or lobectomy (six cases), resection of a segment of small intestine (three cases), brain biopsy at craniotomy (two cases), nephrectomy (one case), biopsy of an ischiorectal mass (one case), and biopsy of a parametrial mass (one case).

The classical sequence of events in choriocarcinoma is a gestation in some form followed by abnormal vaginal bleeding, then a curettage for diagnosis; before chemotherapy, a positive diagnosis on curettings was almost invariably followed by hysterectomy, usually with bilateral salpingo-oophorectomy. In this series, the classical sequence occurred in only 39 (40%) of the 96 cases of gestational choriocarcinoma, but in only nine instances was hysterectomy not performed after a positive curettage. Both curettings and hysterectomy were positive for choriocarcinoma in 12 (27%) of the 44 fatal cases of Group I and in 26 (62%) of the 42 nonfatal cases of Group IV. Of these 42 nonfatal cases, in 35 there was a hysterectomy, and in only one instance was the uterus negative for choriocarcinoma following a positive curettage.

In patients who succumb to choriocarcinoma, no primary lesion may be found in the uterus. In 15 of the 44 autopsied cases, hysterectomy had not been performed. Of these 15, in nine cases there was no tumor in the uterus at autopsy; in three cases choriocarcinoma was present; in two cases a scarred or necrotic mass was presumed to be evidence of privious tumor; and in one case a small nodule of choriocarcinoma in the myometrium and an endometrium free of tumor was found. In all, 72 of the 96 patients with gestational choriocarcinoma underwent hysterectomy at some stage in their disease. Of the 24 patients who did not, 18 died and six survived.

Gross and Microscopical Features

The usual gross configuration of a primary uterine choriocarcinoma (FIGURES 1, 18, 19, 21, 22, & 25) is that of a bulky, infiltrating mass of dark-red tissue, often fungating (FIGURES 22 & 25), occasionally perforating the uterus (FIGURE 18), rarely circumscribed or sharply demarcated from the myometrium (FIGURE 20). The tissue is dark red from hemorrhage; areas of hemorrhagic necrosis usually account for most of the volume of the tumor. The microscopical composition of the tumor is neoplastic cytotrophoblast (CTB) and neoplastic syncitiotrophoblast (STB) without an intrinsic stroma, presenting either as an extensive infiltration of the uterine wall (FIGURE 26) or as a solid mass (FIGURE 23). Invasion of venous channels in the endometrium (FIGURES 24 & 27) and myometrium (FIGURES 26 & 28) is a common feature. Inasmuch as neither the primary nor secondary lesions of choriocarcinoma have their own stroma, blood is supplied from the maternal organ harboring the tumor. Often this blood flows in channels lined by flattened syncitiotrophoblastic cells, resembling those found in the intervillous spaces through which maternal blood circulates in the normal hemorchorial placenta. The absence of stromal support of these channels (FIGURES 17, 29, & 154–156) facilitates the extravasation of blood into adjacent tumor tissue. Therefore, choriocarcinoma is usually described as soft and friable, rarely as fleshy, and hardly ever as solid.

At the junction between tumor and myometrium, in a number of cases (FIGURES 62 & 63) free communications between sheets of neoplasm and patent myometrial veins can be demonstrated, and masses of choriocarcinoma may interdigitate, surround bundles of smooth muscle, or be surrounded by nests of tumor in venous lumina (FIGURES 60 & 64). In some instances, there is a zone of lymphocytic infiltration between the choriocarcinoma and the myometrium

(FIGURES 56 & 57), but this varies in intensity and may be absent (FIGURES 65 & 66), even when venous invasion is present. Elston[27] correlated the intensity of the cellular reaction to choriocarcinoma with survival, and found that an intense response by lymphocytes, plasma cells, and histiocytes is associated with a more favorable response to chemotherapy.

Secondary deposits of choriocarcinoma in all organs tend to be spherical (FIGURES 128, 129, 146–149, 152, 173, & 209). Central hemorrhage and necrosis is usually present; the characteristic microscopical appearance of the "trophoblastic nodule" is that of a thin rim of trophoblast surrounding a center of hemorrhage and necrosis (FIGURES 130, 150, 153, 176, 211, 212, & 254).

In primary uterine choriocarcinoma, the arrangement of trophoblastic elements is usually haphazard and without recognizable pattern. Occasionally, there are areas in which cords or masses of CTB are surrounded by layers of STB in the form of vascular channels (FIGURES 17, 28, & 44), but in no sense can this be interpreted as a pattern of differentiation. The usual random mixture of CTB and STB varies greatly (FIGURES 33–35, 38, 39, 42, 58, & 59). Bizarre cell forms are frequent; the multinucleated "plasmodial masses" of STB assume various sizes and shapes (FIGURES 35 & 38); cytoplasmic vacuoles are numerous.

Absence of molar villi has customarily been used as a criterion to distinguish choriocarcinoma from lesser degrees of trophoblastic disease, especially chorioadenoma destruens. In all cases but one (case 31) in this series, no chorionic villi were found in either curettings or hysterectomy specimens. In case 31, hysterectomy was performed 3 months after the evacuation of a hydatidiform mole (FIGURE 2). Sections from the uterus showed a few molar villi surrounded by broad sheets of proliferated trophoblast invading the myometrium (FIGURES 3 & 4); a diagnosis of chorioadenoma destruens was made at the time. Pulmonary metastases developed, and despite chemotherapy the patient died 17 months after hysterectomy. Postmortem examination revealed extensive pulmonary metastases of trophoblastic tissue without villi, similar metastases in the liver (FIGURE 5), and a large pelvic mass of similar villus-free tissue. The case is considered to be a choriocarcinoma arising from the trophoblast of an invasive hydatidiform mole. Review of English and American literature from 1950 to 1960 yielded 145 cases of adequately documented chorioadenoma destruens; five of these cases died with histologically verified villus-free metastases (3.4%), which seems a reasonable figure for the frequency of the development of choriocarcinoma from an invasive mole. However, as Novak and Seah[9] and others have indicated, the presence of chorionic villi in curettings or hysterectomy specimens is a useful practical criterion for separating less aggressive trophoblastic lesions from choriocarcinoma.

Given adequate sampling and well-prepared sections, problems in histopathological diagnosis of choriocarcinoma rarely arise in the examination of hysterectomy specimens. The presence of vascular invasion by clumps of trophoblast is not a useful criterion for distinguishing choriocarcinoma from chorioadenoma, for it is present in both lesions. Although it is more easily demonstrated in choriocarcinoma and chorioadenoma than in noninvasive moles and the normal placental site, vascular invasion is present to some extent in every pregnancy, as studies of the pulmonary vascular bed of pregnant women have repeatedly shown.

Uterine curettage is almost always diagnostic when choriocarcinoma arises from a term delivery, for there is little difficulty in distinguishing the neoplastic trophoblast of choriocarcinoma from any form of retained trophoblast attendant upon a normal term gestation. However, evaluation of curettings obtained at some interval after the evacuation of a hydatidiform mole may be difficult. If molar villi are present, they may represent either portions of a retained mole or the superficial portion of an invasive mole. If molar villi are not found, the pathologist must be reasonably certain that the tissue supplied is adequate in volume and has been thoroughly sampled and sectioned before venturing upon a diagnosis of choriocarcinoma. In such cases, all material received should be processed, and multiple sections should be examined.

That exuberant reaction at the placental site known as "syncytial endometritis," "postmolar endometritis," or "trophoblastic endometritis" must be distinguished from the lesions in which trophoblast proliferates more actively. When the available anatomical material leaves room for doubt, a policy of conservatism is advocated; in such cases, repeated estimations of the HCG titer may be very useful, and, if bleeding recurs, a second curettage may yield diagnostic material. It is not uncommon to find in curettings some fragments of myometrium infiltrated by trophoblast; this finding does not warrant a diagnosis of choriocarcinoma, for trophoblastic infiltration of the placental site is a constant phenomenon in normal and molar pregnancies. In the latter, a greater degree of trophoblastic infiltration may make the lesion seem more dangerous than it really is. In a number of instances, it may not be possible to make a definitive histopathological diagnosis from the examination of curettings, and their interpretation should always be made in relation to the patient's history.

In cases of choriocarcinoma arising from nonmolar abortions, there may be an unusual degree of trophoblastic proliferation in the curettings obtained at the time of abortion (FIGURES 44 & 45). If bleeding persists, a second curettage usually furnishes material sufficient for definitive diagnosis. In a few patients, the original aborted material consists of nothing but sheets of neoplastic trophoblast without chorionic villi; these may be examples of what has been termed choriocarcinoma *ab initio*.[28]

In three patients in this series, at hysterectomy the choriocarcinoma appeared on examination to be rather superficially engrafted to the lower uterine segment only. All three patients responded favorably to chemotherapy. Conversely, in several instances the primary uterine choriocarcinoma infiltrated the uterine wall so deeply that tumor in continuity extended into the parametrial veins, and there were satellite nodules in the myometrium.

In patients who died after chemotherapy, it was not uncommon to find some completely necrotic metastases (FIGURES 168 & 169) and metastases with viable trophoblast in other vital organs. In two cases of Group V (cases 97, 98), the primary uterine tumor was entirely necrotic, with no viable trophoblast in multiple sections; both patients had had numerous courses of chemotherapy.

The distribution of metastases in fatal, autopsied cases is summarized in TABLE 6 and in nonfatal cases in TABLE 7. The principal loci for secondary deposits are the lungs, brain, and liver. Some features merit special attention: Massive hemoperitoneum from ruptured hepatic metastasis was observed in five cases. The single case in which a tumor embolus was found in a branch of a coronary artery (FIGURE 220) showed a small healing myocardial infarct (FIGURE 221). In the single example of metastasis to the mammary gland (FIGURE 244), there was diffuse lobular hyperplasia abutting the tumor but not elsewhere in the gland. In metastases to bone (FIGURE 235), the surrounding marrow was depleted of myelopoietic elements, possible evidence of local competition for folate, for the marrow elsewhere was not depressd. Hematognous metastasis is the rule in choriocarcinoma, and it is somewhat surprising to find tumor deposits

TABLE 6

DISTRIBUTION OF METASTASES IN AUTOPSIED CASES (GROUPS I AND III)

Location of Metastasis	Group I (44 Cases)	Group III (4 Cases)
Lung		
Viable	42	2
Necrotic	2	
Liver	26	3
Brain	28*	1
Kidneys	21	1
Spleen		
Viable	10	2
Necrotic	1	
Emboli only	2	
Small intestine	12	2
Large intestine	1	
Stomach	4	
Pancreas	3	1
Vagina	9	1
Adrenal gland	4	
Thyroid gland	3	1
Skin	2	
Salivary gland	1	
Gingiva	1	
Right ovary	1	
Breast	1	
Heart	4	
Ascending aorta	1	
Main pulmonary artery	1	
Bone	3	
Peritoneum	4	2
Diaphragm	3	1
Pelvic soft tissue	6	2
Peripheral veins	2	
Skeletal muscle	3	
Lymph nodes (tertiary)	7	1
Chest wall	2	
Positive chest roentgenogram	39	2

*Including one case of cerebral hemorrhage without identified trophoblast.

in lymph nodes in seven cases (FIGURES 231–233). But these lymph nodes all drained organs with secondary deposits of choriocarcinoma and might be construed as containing tertiary deposits. Moreover, lymph nodes do have blood supplies, and an interpretation of tertiary deposition cannot be asserted with certainty. The distribution of metastases in the four cases of primary ovarian nongestational choriocarcinoma follow those expected for ovarian neoplasms.

The paucity of histologically verified metastases in the 42 nonfatal cases of gestational choriocarcinoma (TABLE 7) is in conformity with these patients' fortunate clinical course. In this group, a single pulmonary metastasis was resected at thoracotomy for a coin lesion 8 months after a hydatidiform mole. More than three-fourths of the patients who survived had roentgenographic evidence of pulmonary metastases.

TABLE 7

SECONDARY LESIONS IN NONFATAL CASES (GROUP IV)*

Lesion	No. of Cases
Vaginal nodules	7
Ischiorectal area	1
Scalp	1
Lungs (intravascular emboli)	1
Positive chest roentgenograms	30

*Total number of cases, 42.

Vaginal nodules of choriocarcinoma develop from retrograde spread of neoplastic trophoblast embolic from the uterus into the paravaginal venous plexus. In some instances, the tumor remains intravascular (FIGURE 85), but in others it invades the adjacent soft parts (FIGURES 87 & 88). Vaginal nodules also occur in association with uncomplicated hydatidiform moles as well as with chorioadenoma destruens and choriocarcinoma. In one patient (case 4), the presenting symptom was a vaginal nodule (FIGURE 85) 1 month after term delivery; the hysterectomy specimen showed no tumor in the uterus. Vaginal nodules often ulcerate and may be the source of severe bleeding, which is sometimes difficult to control by local measures. Their presence or absence has slight prognostic value, for their occurrence in fatal cases (nine out of 46) is not significantly different from their occurrence in nonfatal cases (seven out of 42).

Endocrine Pathology

The endocrine status of a patient with choriocarcinoma may be described as pseudopregnancy; HCG, elaborated in large amounts, produces characteristic changes in a number of target organs. These changes vary greatly from case to case, but the tissues studied in this series had been exposed to high circulating titers. The variation in response of target organs cannot be attributed to exposure to only slight or moderate amounts of HCG, for surgical specimens were obtained when urinary titers were high, and almost all patients who came to autopsy had titers of 30,000 or more mouse units shortly before death. The changes seen in target organs are as follows:

Cervix Uteri. At least one section of the uterine cervix was available for study in 90 cases. In two instances, there was focal atypism of the stratified squamous epithelium of the exocervix. In one patient, the lesion consisted of a sharply demarcated zone of squamous cells with ballooned, clear cytoplasm and shrunken, pyknotic nuclei (FIGURE 82); there was only trivial inflammation in the underlying stroma. In the other patient, there was diffuse atypical metaplasia of squamous cells with basal cell hyperplasia (FIGURE 83) extending over the exocervix and into the gland-like endocervical clefts (FIGURE 84); underlying the epithelial surface was a diffuse chronic inflammatory exudate. Similar epithelial alterations have been described in biopsies taken during pregnancy; they are not specific for pregnancy, for comparable lesions can be seen in the cervices of nonpregnant women, albeit less frequently. Ectopic decidual reactions were not seen in the endocervical stroma in any of the sections reviewed. Some degree of hypersecretion and inspissation of endocervical mucus was present in almost every hysterectomy specimen examined; it was not seen in the cervix at autopsy.

Endometrium. Conventionally, endometrium associated with choriocarcinoma exhibits a decidual reaction, which is regularly present whether the choriocarcinoma is uterine or extrauterine only. Although the decidual lining may be edematous and thick, it commonly is not appreciably thicker than ordinary endometrium in the late secretory phase. When present, decidual reactions ranged from the intense and diffuse (FIGURES 24 & 27) to the weak, patchy, and even focal (FIGURES 70 & 73). In 38 cases, the presence or absence of a decidual reaction could not be determined, for the endometrium in the material available had been entirely replaced by tumor. The following observations are based on 62 cases.

Uterine curettings positive for choriocarcinoma had some degree of decidual reaction in 18 cases and no decidual reaction in ten. A similar ratio was observed in hysterectomy specimens; 17 contained decidual reactions of varying degrees, and seven did not. But decidual reactions were very few in material obtained at autopsy. In 16 autopsy specimens suitable for study, the endometrium was thin and atrophic in 11; there were weak decidual reactions in two (FIGURES 73, 74); there was a secretory endometrium (both associated with hydatidiform moles) in two (FIGURES 71, 72) and there was an endometrial pattern similar to that produced by estrogen-progestagen preparations in one unusual instance (FIGURES 76–78).

In 50 cases in which suitable material was available from both the endometrium and the ovaries, an endometrial decidual reaction was present in 17, of which eight had a concomitant ectopic ovarian decidual reaction (FIGURES 114–116); 33 uteri showed no decidual change, but ten of these had ectopic ovarian decidual reactions. An unusual ectopic decidual reaction was seen in parametrial soft tissue (FIGURES 80 & 81) adjacent to an infiltrating uterine choriocarcinoma. Ectopic decidua was found as frequently in autopsy specimens as in surgical specimens.

A striking feature of the decidual reaction in patients with choriocarcinoma is the failure of spiral arteries to develop as they do in the normal menstrual cycle. In this respect, the spiral arteries are unlike those seen in normal pregnancy and resemble those present in the uteri of patients treated by cyclical oral administration of synthetic estrogen-progestagen preparations; a good example is case 57 (FIGURE 75), in which dilated venules were prominent. Sometimes the endometrium in the presence of choriocarcinoma does not respond at all; endometrium adjacent to choriocarcinoma may be inert (FIGURE 67) or, in fields some distance from tumor, show only slight loosening of the stroma (FIGURE 68).

Two of the four patients with nongestational choriocarcinoma could be evaluated with respect to endometrium. In case 46, the endometrium was in the early secretory phase without decidual reaction when laparotomy disclosed an ovarian tumor composed of choriocarcinoma and dysgerminoma and a liver containing extensive metastatic choriocarcinoma, later confirmed at autopsy (FIGURES 128 & 129). In case 47, the endometrium of a 9-year-old girl with ovarian teratocarcinoma containing choriocarcinomatous elements was slightly thickened but showed no mitoses, secretion, or decidual transformation (FIGURE 137). Atypical epithelial configurations of endometrial glands (FIGURE 79) as described by Arias-Stella[29] were identified in six of 62 specimens in which the endometrium was suitable for examination.

Ovaries. The characteristic reaction of the ovaries to the presence of a hydatidiform mole or a gonadotropin-secreting tumor is bilateral enlargement by theca-lutein cysts. Of the 96 cases of gestational choriocarcinoma, sections from one or both ovaries were available for study in 50. In three of the remaining 46 cases in which the ovaries were not available, there was information that at laparotomy the ovaries appeared large and cystic.

In 32 of the 50 cases in which the ovary could be studied, a theca-lutein reaction was present; in 18 cases, it was absent in the presence of high HCG titers. The theca-lutein reactions varied considerably. In a few instances, the ovaries contained multiple cysts, up to 1.5 cm in diameter, with inner linings of luteinized granulosa surrounded by an outer mantle of luteinized theca interna (FIGURES 94, 95); this configuration was most common during the 6-month interval after evacuation of a hydatidiform mole. A more common finding was the presence of small cysts a few millimeters in diameter lined by a relatively thin layer of luteinized theca interna (FIGURES 96 & 97), scattered nests of luteinized theca cells at the periphery of an atretic follicle (FIGURE 112), or small groups of luteinized theca cells lying here and there in the cortical stroma (FIGURE 113). In occasional instances, a persistently elevated HCG titer following a hydatidiform mole could preserve a corpus luteum of pregnancy for 2 years (FIGURE 98), but usually theca-lutein cysts and luteinized stroma were absent after such an interval (FIGURE 99). It should be emphasized that luteinization of granulosa cells lining a graafian follicle occurs only in the formation of a normal corpus luteum menstruationis, in trophoblastic disease, and in patients receiving large doses of exogenous pituitary gonadotropin; luteinization is confined to theca interna and and cortical stroma in those endocrine disorders characterized by anovulation, virilization, and related phenomena. Occasional unusual ovarian configurations were seen; for example, in case 66 the ovary at laparotomy 10 weeks postpartum showed a pattern similar to that seen in the micropolycystic ovary syndrome (FIGURE 101) in the presence of a regressing corpus luteum gestationis.

A lesser degree of luteinization was present in material from autopsies. The changes ranged from scattered expansion of follicles with mild luteinization of theca interna (and occasional plaques of ectopic decidua) (FIGURE 100), to examples in which corpora lutea were found (FIGURES 102, 103) without other evidence of ovarian response. These latter ovaries resembled those of normally menstruating women. In a few cases, the ovary at autopsy could be described as almost inactive (FIGURES 104, 105 & 108), consisting chiefly of medullar corpora albicantia, minimal expansion of graafian follicles, and a bland cortex without luteinization (in these cases, a few plaques of ectopic decidua were sometimes present). In several instances, degenerative changes consisting of calcospherites (FIGURES 109–111) were seen in areas of luteinization. The variable and focal nature of ovarian response, when present, is illustrated by case 57, in which hysterectomy and bilateral salpingo-oophorectomy were performed 1 year after term delivery. The uterus contained choriocarcinoma, and the HCG titer was high. Both ovaries were enlarged and showed a polycystic pattern, and the cysts were lined by prominent layers of theca interna (FIGURE 108); at one point in one cystic follicle there was focal luteinization of granulosa cells (FIGURES 106 & 107).

The presence of ectopic ovarian decidua has already been described in conjunction with the decidual reaction in endometrium. Ectopic decidual plaques (FIGURES 114–116) were present in 18 of the 50 cases studied. The plaques were similar to those seen in normal pregnancy and in those few cases in which ectopic ovarian decidua has occurred in the absence of pregnancy. The ectopic decidual reaction is not the direct result of HCG stimulation; it is a reaction of subcoelomic mesenchymal tissue, embryologically cognate with endometrial stroma and usually inconspicuous in the adult, to estrogen priming and progesterone stimulation. Comparable reactions can be induced by administration of synthetic progrestagens in high dosage. It is generally thought that ectopic ovarian decidua occurs only in the presence of amounts of ovarian steroid hormones in excess of the amounts present during the normal menstrual cycle, but analysis of the urinary metabolites of endogenous ovarian hormones in women with choriocarcinoma have failed to support this hypothesis.

In five cases, examination of the ovarian hilus revealed a moderate degree of hilus cell hyperplasia in the form of prominent nests of medium-sized polyhedral cells with dark eosinophilic cytoplasm (FIGURE 117), often associated with nerve fibers (FIGURE 118). Lipochrome pigment was identified in these cells, but crystalloids of Reincke were not. This observation is consistent with the report by Segaloff and his associates[30] that a single injection of HCG in adult women will elicit hilus cell hyperplasia. Most of the sections of ovary examined did not provide adequate sampling from the hilar region, and this hyperplasia may be more frequent than these observations would suggest. Metastasis of choriocarcinoma to the ovary was found in one instance (case 34). Neither the ovary with the metastasis nor the contralateral ovary showed theca-lutein cysts, stromal luteinization, ectopic decidua, or hilus cell hyperplasia (FIGURES 119 & 120).

The four nongestational choriocarcinomas arising in complex primary ovarian tumors merit illustration of their uncommon morphology and descriptions of the contralateral ovaries. Case 48 was a mixture of separate elements of choriocarcinoma and disgerminoma (FIGURES 138–140). The contralateral ovary was stated to be grossly and microscopically normal, but sections for study were not available. Case 45 was an embryonal carcinoma with choriocarcinomatous elements (FIGURES 121 & 122); the contralateral ovary contained many cystically dilated follicles (FIGURE 123), but there was no evidence of theca-lutein reaction or stromal luteinization. In case 52, a mixture of choriocarcinoma and disgerminoma (FIGURES 124–132), the contralateral ovary was not present. The patient had never menstruated, and it is considered likely that the tumor arose in a dysgenetic gonad; extensive metastases consisted of choriocarcinoma only. In case 53, a teratocarcinoma with choriocarcinomatous elements in a 9-year-old girl (FIGURES 133 & 134), the contralateral ovary contained many cystically expanded follicles lined by nonluteinized granulosa cells (FIGURE 135), but the theca interna showed only minimal accentuation; hyperplasia of ovarian hilar cells was present (FIGURE 136).

Mammary Gland. Tissue from this organ was available for study only from the 48 autopsied cases. In nine instances, the mammary lobules were hyperplastic; the hyperplasia involved ductules, terminal lobules, and intralobular stroma (FIGURES 245–250). Ectasia of the major ducts was also present (FIGURES 245 & 246). In three instances, small secretory vacuoles were present in the cytoplasm of terminal lobular cells (FIGURES 248).

In one patient (case 21), a 48-year-old woman, an infiltrating duct cell carcinoma, less than 1.0 cm in diameter, was found at autopsy; mild lobular and ductal hyperplasia were present elsewhere in the breast. In another patient (case 2), local excision of choriocarcinoma metastatic to the breast was performed 18 months after term delivery. Mild lobular hyperplasia was present in the immediate vicinity of the metastasis, but tissue more than 1 cm away from it was normal. When this patient died 8 months later with persistent choriocarcinoma (but no more metastases in the breasts), there was no hyperplasia in tissue removed from either breast at autopsy.

Adrenal Glands. The adrenal glands were examined in the 48 autopsied cases. In four cases (of the 44 in Group I), metastases were present (FIGURES 254–257). No changes of an endocrine nature were detected. Specifically, there was no hyperplasia of the zones of the adrenal cortex. and no medullary lesions were encountered. Narrowing of the cortex and depletion of cortical lipids, changes commonly found at autopsy in patients dying after prolonged, debilitating illness, irrespective of cause, were present.

Thyroid Gland. The thyroid gland was examined in the 48 autopsied cases. Metastases were present in three of 44 cases of gestational choriocarcinoma and in one of the four cases of nongestational choriocarcinoma (FIGURES 251 & 252). Although clinical and laboratory evidence of hyperthyroidism had been present in five of the 44 cases in Group I,[31] treatment had made them euthyroid at the time of autopsy, and residual traces of antecedent hyperfunction were not detected. Focal follicular hyperplasia (FIGURE 253) was seen at autopsy in one methimazole-treated patient (case 19), and in two others (cases 23 and 29) there was microscopical evidence of involution following recent antecedent hyperplasia. In addition to these patients, two patients had nontoxic nodules, one had a follicular adenoma, and one had a history of carcinoma of the thyroid gland treated by surgery and radioiodine 8 years previously; no carcinoma was found in the scarred, atrophic gland at autopsy. In Group III, apart from the single case with metastasis, no changes were found.

Islets of Langerhans. In eight of the 44 cases in Group I, a mild degree of hyperplasia of the islets of Langerhans was found. The hyperplasia was limited to areas in the body and tail of the pancreas, where the islets were more numerous, larger, and more cellular (FIGURES 190–192). In one patient (case 28), a small (8-mm) islet cell adenoma was present (FIGURE 189). Clinically, no patient was noted to suffer from hypoglycemic episodes, and all blood sugar determinations were normal. Metastasis to the pancreas was found in three cases (FIGURE 188), but in none of these was there hyperplasia of the islets.

Adenohypophysis. At least one section of pituitary gland was available for study in the 48 autopsied cases. The HCG titer was elevated in all of these patients shortly before death. No consistent pattern of altered cell populations was found. Pregnancy changes were not encountered. Aseptic necrosis was present in the adenohypophyses of three patients (cases 25, 29, and 38), never involving more than half of the lobe (FIGURES 258–261). Cerebral metastases were present in all three cases, and the necrosis probably was caused by changes in intracranial pressure and the hemodynamics to the hypothalamic region.

Pharmacopathology

The toxic clinical and pathological manifestations associated with antifolic and other antimetabolic oncolytic drugs are well known, both with respect to the nature and distribution of lesions. Some degree of clinical toxicity was noted in all of the treated patients in this series. The 48 autopsied cases (Groups I and III) included six patients who had received less than one full course of chemotherapy. Major lesions ascribable to drug toxicity were found in 24 cases. Residual viable choriocarcinoma was found at autopsy in 46 (all but two) cases. In some instances, it is difficult to estimate the importance of toxic lesions as causes of death, but if the hazards of chemotherapy are to be appreciated, some evaluation of the drug-induced lesions is essential. In many patients who died with both metastatic choriocarcinoma and toxic lesions, drug dosage had been increased because of persistent (or resistant) tumor. Eight of the 24 patients with severe toxic lesions at autopsy were admitted with far-advanced, widely disseminated choriocarcinoma and died after two courses or less of methotrexate. At the other extereme are a patient who died after 16 courses of methotrexate and another patient who died after ten courses of methotrexate, two courses of vincaleukoblastine, five courses of actinomycin D, three courses of actinomycin D plus chlorambucil, and three courses of "triple therapy" (methotrexate, chlorambucil, and actinomycin D).

The anatomical lesions associated with drug toxicity and the illustrations of these lesions in this series are listed in TABLE 8. Lesions principally involved the liver, kidney, bone marrow, and portions of the gastrointestinal tract. Lesions of the tongue, epiglottis, esophagus, and lower gastrointestinal tract were usually pseudomembranous, and it was not uncommon to see colonies of bacteria in the underlying blood vessels.

TABLE 8

DISTRIBUTION OF ANATOMICAL LESIONS ASSOCIATED WITH DRUG TOXICITY

Location of Lesion	Type	No. of Cases	Illustration Nos.
Liver	Fatty metamorphosis	6	FIGURES 184–186
	Toxic hepatitis (fat plus necrosis)	2	FIGURE 187
	Posthepatic cirrhosis	2	FIGURE 183
Gastrointestinal tract	Ulcerative lesions	9	FIGURES 206–208
	Necrotizing glossitis	3	FIGURE 202
	Necrotizing esophagitis	3	FIGURES 203–205
	Rupture of esophagus (persistent vomiting)	1	FIGURE 195
	Necrotizing epiglottitis	2	FIGURES 262–264
Kidney	Renal hemorrhage	3	FIGURES 215–217
Bone marrow	Toxic depression	8	FIGURES 237–243
		39	

A significant number of patients died with (and probably of) terminal sepsis. Of these 12 infections, there were one instance of peritonitis, one of staphylococcal enteritis, one of staphylococcal pneumonia, two of gas gangrene, and seven of bacteremia, including two with *Pseudomonas aeruginosa,* two with *Staphylococcus aureus,* one with Friedlander's bacillus, and two with mixed infections (one with a combination of *Escherichia coli, S. aureus,* and Friedlander's bacillus and one with a combination of *P. aeruginosa, S. aureus,* and *Monilia*). The latter was the only patient in the series with a terminal mycosis, a distinct contrast to current experience with patients dying in the course of chemotherapy of leukemias and lymphomas. Morphological evidence of sepsis was present in several forms, the most notable being microabscesses in soft tissue associated with gram-negative bacillus bacteremia (FIGURE 271), and the demonstration of *Clostridium perfringens* in the lung (FIGURE 272) and in other tissues of patients dying with gas gangrene.

A particularly impressive example of the hazards of chemotherapy is case 37, a 47-year-old woman who was diagnosed as having choriocarcinoma 4 months after a spontaneous abortion. Hysterectomy and bilateral salpingo-oophorectomy were done promptly, but within 3 months a vaginal nodule appeared, followed by hematuria from a renal metastasis that was treated by nephrectomy. A single course of methotrexate begun the day after nephrectomy led to agranulocytosis and death from bacteremia 3 weeks later. Although a thrombus of choriocarcinoma in the left iliac vein persisted, the few small pulmonary metastases were completely necrotic but surrounded by colonies of bacteria (FIGURE 169).

Of the 24 patients with drug-induced toxic lesions, all had received methotrexate; ten had received no other antitumor drug. Five patients received courses of a *Vinca* alkaloid (either leukoblastine or leukocristine); eight were treated with courses of actinomycin D alone, two with actinomycin D in combination with chlorambucil, six with "triple therapy" (methotrexate, actinomycin D, and chlorambucil), and a minority of patients had received nitrogen mustard, cyclophosphamide, x-irradiation, and other drugs at one stage or another. Since the anatomical lesions of toxicity are all similar in nature and distribution, analysis of the pathological material does not permit any conclusion as to which lesions might be expected after any specific drug. However, the patient who received x-ray therapy died with significant pulmonary fibrosis. The two examples of posthepatitic cirrhosis cannot be attributed to the drug therapy, for the probability of "needle" hepatitis in patients with prolonged hospitalization is great. However, it should be noted that even small amounts of methotrexate can produce lesions detectable at autopsy. Two patients admitted with widely disseminated choriocarcinoma who failed to survive even one full course of methotrexate had ulcerative lesions of the mouth, esophagus, and large intestine; one of them died of staphylococcal septicemia. Another complication of chemotherapy is rupture of a necrotic tumor with massive hemorrhage. Five patients died of massive hemoperitoneum from ruptured hepatic metastases.

Acknowledgments

The authors gratefully acknowledge the unfailing patience and wise counsel of Harold L. Stewart, M.D., formerly Director of the Laboratory of Pathology of the National Cancer Institute, who encouraged us to initiate and complete this study. We also wish to extend our sincere thanks to Mr. Gebhardt Gsell, formerly photographer in the Laboratory of Pathology at the National Cancer Institute, whose great technical skill was responsible for the illustrations shown in this paper.

References

1. Ober, W. B., Ed. 1959. Trophoblast and Its Tumors. Ann N.Y. Acad. Sci. **80**(1): 1–284.
2. Teacher, J. H. 1903. On chorionepithelioma and the occurrence of chorionepitheliomatous and hydatidiform mole-like structures in teratomata. J. Obstet. Gynaec. Brit. Emp. **4**: 1–64 & 145–199.
3. Park, W. W. & J. C. Lees. 1950. Choriocarcinoma. Arch. Path. **49**: 73–104 & 205–241.

4. BENIRSCHKE, K. & S. G. DRISCOLL. 1967. The Pathology of the Human Placenta. Springer-Verlag. New York, N.Y.
5. HERTIG, A. T. 1968. Human Trophoblast. Charles C Thomas, Publ. Springfield, Ill.
6. BAGSHAWE, K. D. 1969. Choriocarcinoma: The Clinical Biology of the Trophoblast and Its Tumours. Edwin Arnold. London, England.
7. HERTZ, R., D. M. BERGENSTAL, M. B. LIPSETT, E. B. PRICE, JR. & T. F. HILBISH. 1958. Chemotherapy of choriocarcinoma and related trophoblastic tumors in women. J.A.M.A. **168**: 845–854.
8. PARK, W. W. 1967. Clinical Choriomatosis. Proc. Roy. Soc. Med. **60**: 235–240.
9. NOVAK, E. & C. S. SEAH. 1954. Choriocarcinoma of the uterus. Amer. J. Obstet. Gynec. **67**: 933–961.
10. HOU, P. C. & S. C. PANG. 1956. Chorionepithelioma: An analytic study of 28 necropsied cases with special reference to the possibility of spontaneous regression. J. Path. Bact. **72**: 95–104.
11. SMALBRAAK, J .1957. Trophoblastic Growths. Elsevier. Amsterdam, The Netherlands.
12. LI, M. C., R. HERTZ & D. B. SPENCER. 1956. Effect of methotrexate therapy upon choriocarcinoma and chorioadenoma. Proc. Soc. Exp. Biol. Med. **93**: 361–366.
13. HERTZ, R., J. LEWIS, JR. & M. B. LIPSETT. 1961. Five years' experience with the chemotherapy of metastatic choriocarcinoma and related trophoblastic tumors in women. Amer. J. Obstet. Gynec. **82**: 631–640.
14. KLINEFELTER, JR., H. F., F. ALBRIGHT & G. C. GRISWOLD. 1943. Experience with quantitative test for normal or decreased amounts of follicle-stimulating hormone in endocrinologic diagnosis. J. Clin. Endocr. **3**: 529–544.
15. SCHOEN, I., B. E. KONWALER & E. NOVAK. 1954. The sex incidence of the fetus or child in maternal choriocarcinoma. Amer. J. Obstet. Gynec. **67**: 1134–1138.
16. PARK, W. W. 1957. The occurrence of sex-chromatin in chorionepitheliomas and hydatidiform moles. J. Path. Bact. **74**: 197–206.
17. CLEMMER, J. J. & G. H. HANSMANN. 1935. The origin of chorionepitheliomas and of emboli from trophoblastic fragments enclosed in the myometrium. Amer. J. Obstet. Gynec. **29**: 526–534.
18. DRISCOLL, S. G. 1963. Choriocarcinoma: An "incidental finding" in a term placenta. Obstet. Gynec. **21**: 96–101.
19. BREWER, J. I. & A. B. GERBIE. 1966. Early development of choriocarcinoma. Amer. J. Obstet. Gynec. **94**: 692–710.
20. MACRAE, D. J. 1951. Chorionepithelioma occurring during pregnancy. J. Obstet. Gynaec. Brit. Emp. **58**: 373–380.
21. BUCKELL, E. W. C. & T. K. OWEN. 1954. Chorionepithelioma in moth and infant. J. Obstet. Gynaec. Brit. Emp. **61**: 329–330.
22. MERCER, R. D., A. C. LAMMERT, R. ANDERSON & J. B. HAZARD. 1958. Choriocarcinoma in mother and infant. J.A.M.A. **166**: 482–483.
23. EVERSON, T. C. & W. H. COLE. 1966. Spontaneous Regression of Cancer. W. B. Saunders Co. Philadelphia, Pa.
24. BARDAWIL, W. A., A. T. HERTIG & J. T. VELARDO. 1957. Regression of trophoblast. I. Hydatidiform mole; a case of unusual features, possibly metastasis and regression; review of literature. Obstet. Gynec. **10**: 614–625.
25. BAGSHAWE, K. D. & C. E. WILDE. 1964. Infusion therapy for pelvic trophoblastic tumors. J. Obstet. Gynaec. Brit. Comm. **71**: 565–572.
26. WIDER, J. A., J. R. MARSHALL, C. W. BARDIN, M. B. LIPSETT & G. ROSS. 1969. Sustained remissions after chemotherapy for primary ovarian cancers containing choriocarcinoma. New Eng. J. Med. **280**: 1439–1442.
27. ELSTON, C. 1969. Cellular reaction to choriocarcinoma. J. Path. Bact. **97**: 261–268.
28. ACOSTA-SISON, H. 1959. *Ab initio* choriocarcinoma. Obstet. Gynec. **13**: 350–352.
29. ARIAS-STELLA, J. 1959. A topographic study of uterine epithelial atypia associated with chorionic tissue. Cancer **12**: 782–790.

30. Segaloff, A., W. H. Sternberg & C. J. Gaskill. 1953. Influence of chorionic gonadotropin on human ovarian hilus cells. J. Clin. Endocr. 13: 139–153.
31. Odell, W. D., R. W. Bates, R. S. Rivlin, M. B. Lipsett & R. Hertz. 1963. Increased thyroid function without clinical hyperthyroidism in patients with choriocarcinoma. J. Clin. Endocr. 23: 658–664.

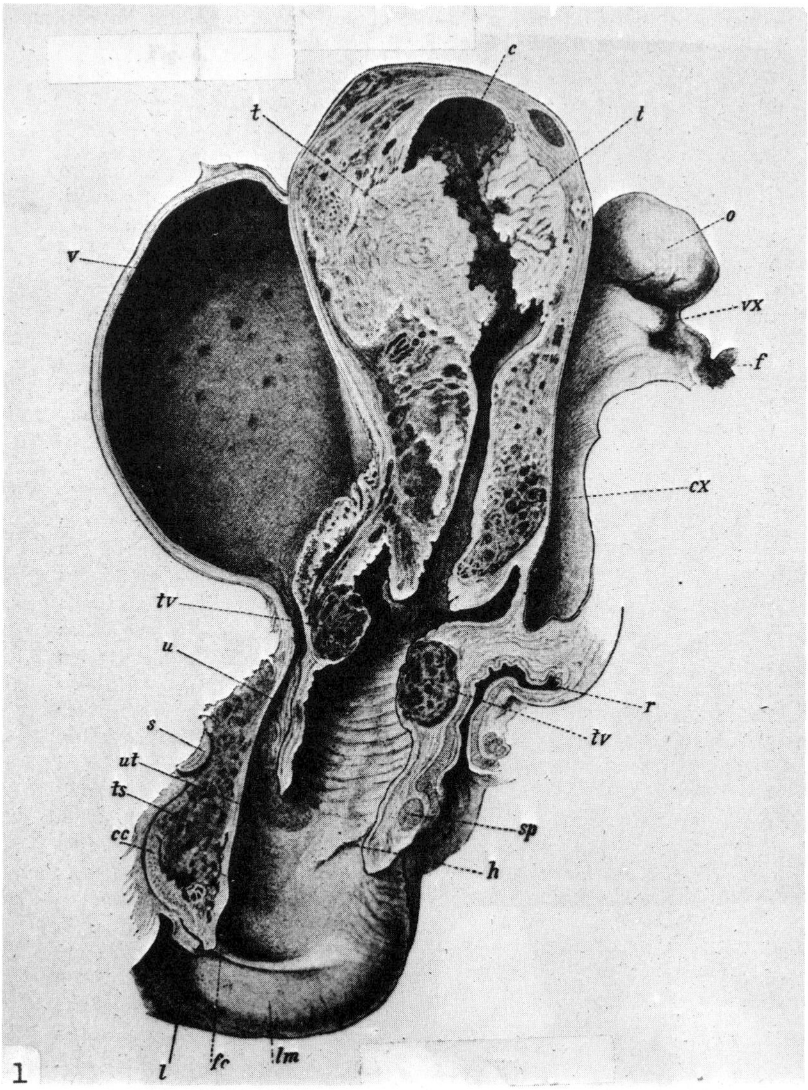

1

FIGURE 1. Sagittal section of pelvic organs, showing a primary choriocarcinoma (t,t) invading the anterior and posterior walls of the uterus, hemorrhagic infiltration of the cervix (cx), and secondary vaginal deposits. (Reproduced from Marchand, F.1898. Über das maligne Chorionepitheliom nebst Mittheilung von 2 neuen Fällen. Z. Geburtsh. Gynaek. 39: 173–258.)

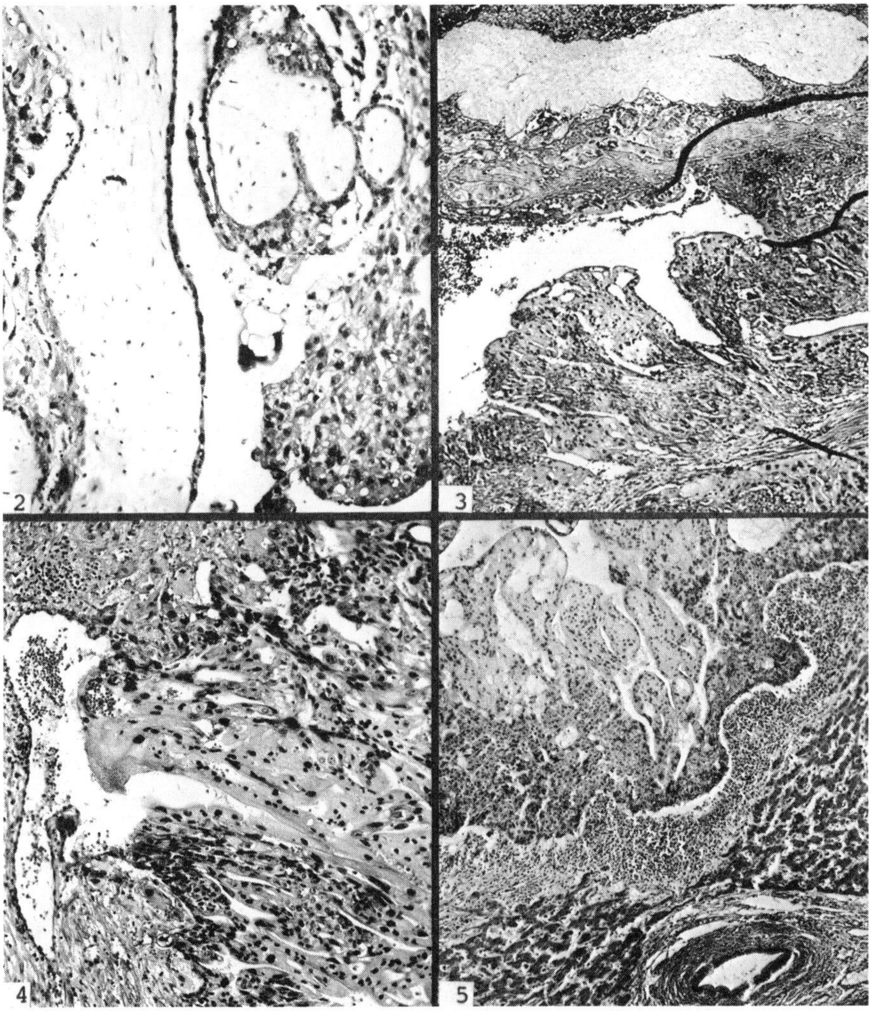

FIGURE 2. *Case 31:* Hydatidiform mole, showing moderate trophoblastic hyperplasia with minimal cellular pleomorphism. (× 100)

FIGURE 3. *Case 31:* Uterus at hysterectomy 13 weeks after a hydatidiform mole, showing a molar villus surrounded by a blood clot and necrotic material, deep to which are sheets of proliferated trophoblast infiltrating the myometrium. (× 55)

FIGURE 4. *Case 31:* Uterus at hysterectomy 13 weeks after a hydatidiform mole, showing proliferated trophoblast invading the myometrium and entering an intramural vein. (× 96)

FIGURE 5. *Case 31:* Liver 20 months after a hydatidiform mole, showing metastatic choriocarcinoma. (× 48)

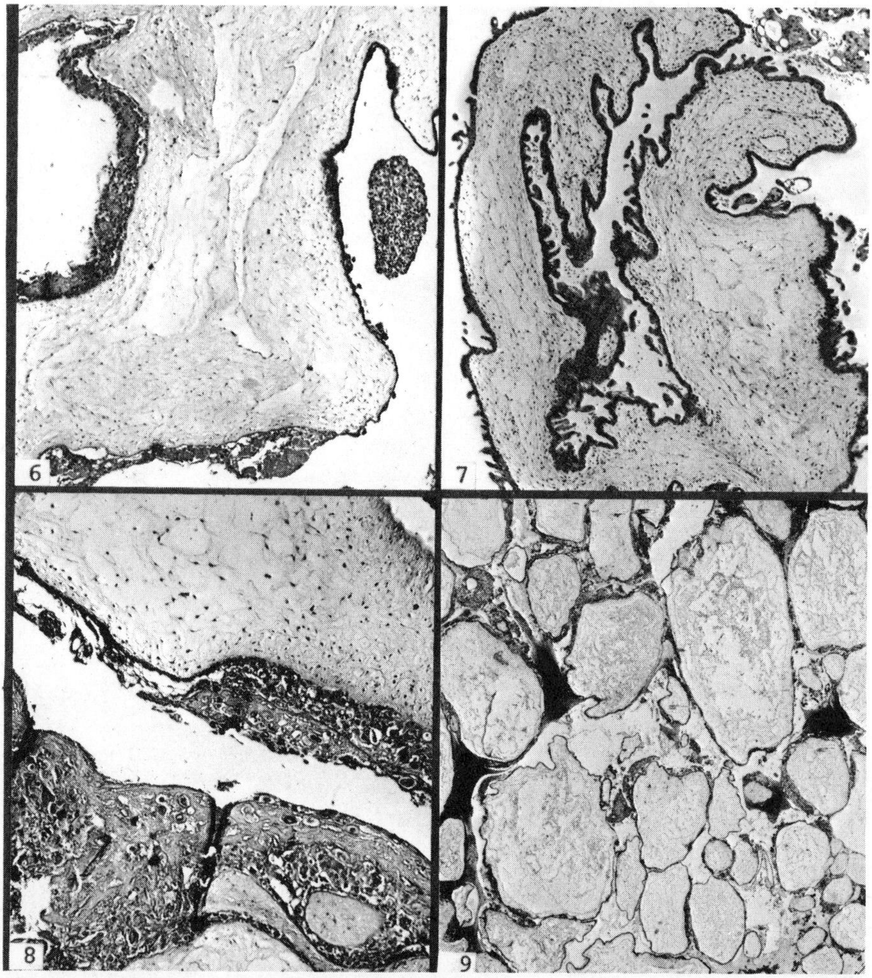

FIGURE 6. *Case 25:* Villus from a hydatidiform mole, showing slight trophoblastic overgrowth. Hysterectomy for choriocarcinoma was performed 18 months later. (× 30)

FIGURE 7. *Case 84:* Villus from a hydatidiform mole, showing moderate trophoblastic overgrowth. Choriocarcinoma was diagnosed at curettage 3 weeks later, following an episode of brisk uterine bleeding. (× 40)

FIGURE 8. *Case 22:* Villi from a hydatidiform mole, showing moderate overgrowth of trophoblast undergoing hyaline degeneration. Choriocarcinoma was diagnosed at hysterectomy 4 months later. (× 48)

FIGURE 9. *Case 33:* Hydatidiform mole at low magnification. Molar villi are mostly covered by thin layers of trophoblast with only moderate overgrowth. (× 9)

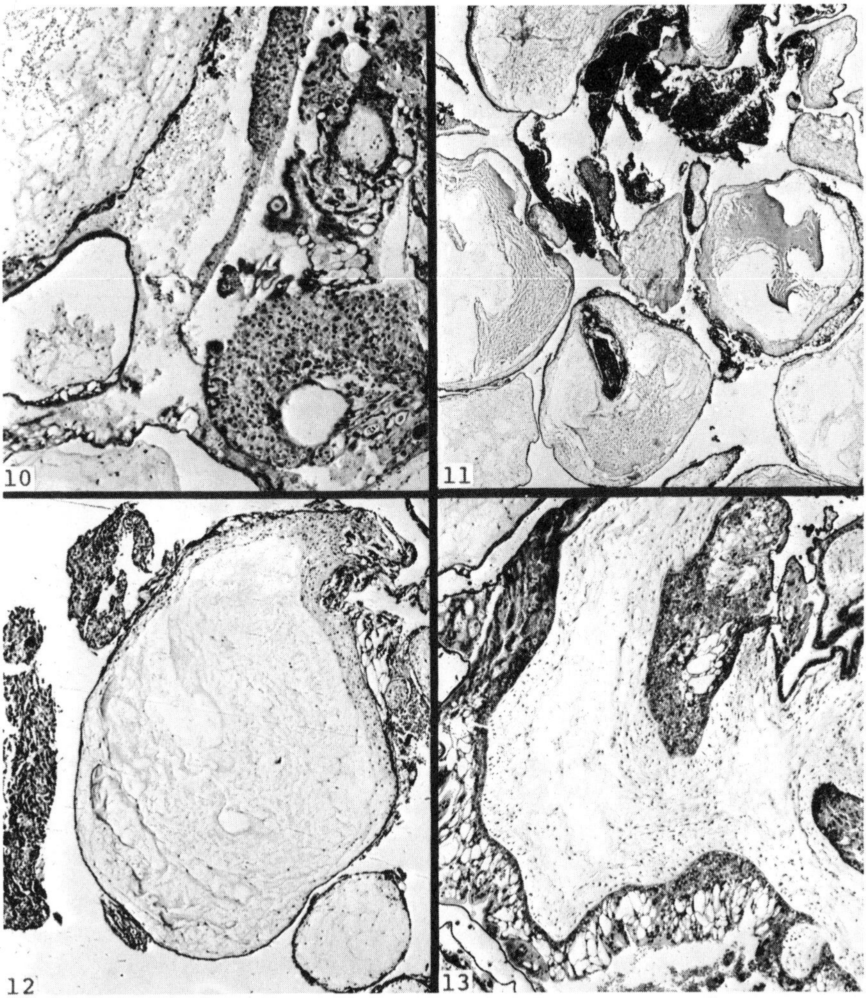

FIGURE 10. *Case 33:* Detail of another area of the mole shown in FIGURE 9, showing maximal degree of trophoblastic overgrowth demonstrable. (× 48) No evidence of trophoblastic disease was found for over 2 years after the mole. Chest x-ray showed bilateral nodules 30 months after the mole, and tissue diagnosis of choriocarcinoma made at laparotomy 5 months later.

FIGURE 11. *Case 98:* Hydatidiform mole, showing pronounced cavitation of the avascular villi and slight trophoblastic overgrowth. (× 12)

FIGURE 12. *Case 98:* Detail of another area of the mole shown in FIGURE 11, demonstrable. (× 35) No viable trophoblast was found in the uterine tumor at hysterectomy performed after extensive chemotherapy. (This case is classified as "probable" choriocarcinoma.)

FIGURE 13. *Case 49:* Hydatidiform mole, showing marked hyperplasia and atypia of trophoblast. (× 44)

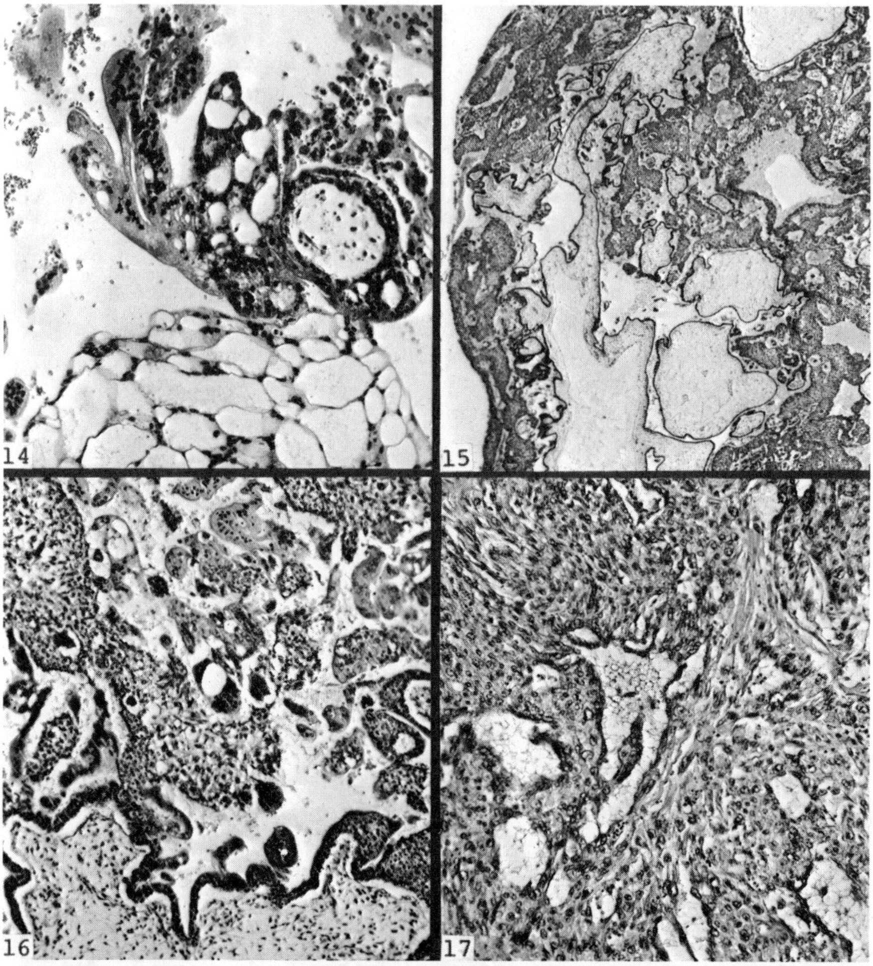

FIGURE 14. *Case 49:* Detail of the mole shown in FIGURE 13, showing bizarre syncytiotrophoblast with nuclear pleomorphism and cytoplasmic vacuolation. (× 76) Curettage 1 year later yielded tissue strongly suggestive of choriocarcinoma, and death occurred 3 months afterward, with clinical and radiological evidence of disseminated neoplasm; autopsy was not permitted.

FIGURE 15. *Case 77:* Hydatidiform mole, showing severe degree of trophoblastic overgrowth. (× 11)

FIGURE 16. *Case 77:* Detail of FIGURE 15, showing surface of a molar villus with sheets of cytotrophoblast and buds of syncytiotrophoblast growing from it. (× 67)

FIGURE 17. *Case 77:* Choriocarcinoma infiltrating uterus at hysterectomy 15 weeks after a hydatidiform mole, showing sheets of cytotrophoblast and sinusoids lined by syncytiotrophoblast mimicking the spatial configuration of the intervillous space in the normal placenta. (× 86) Complete remission was obtained after four courses of methotrexate.

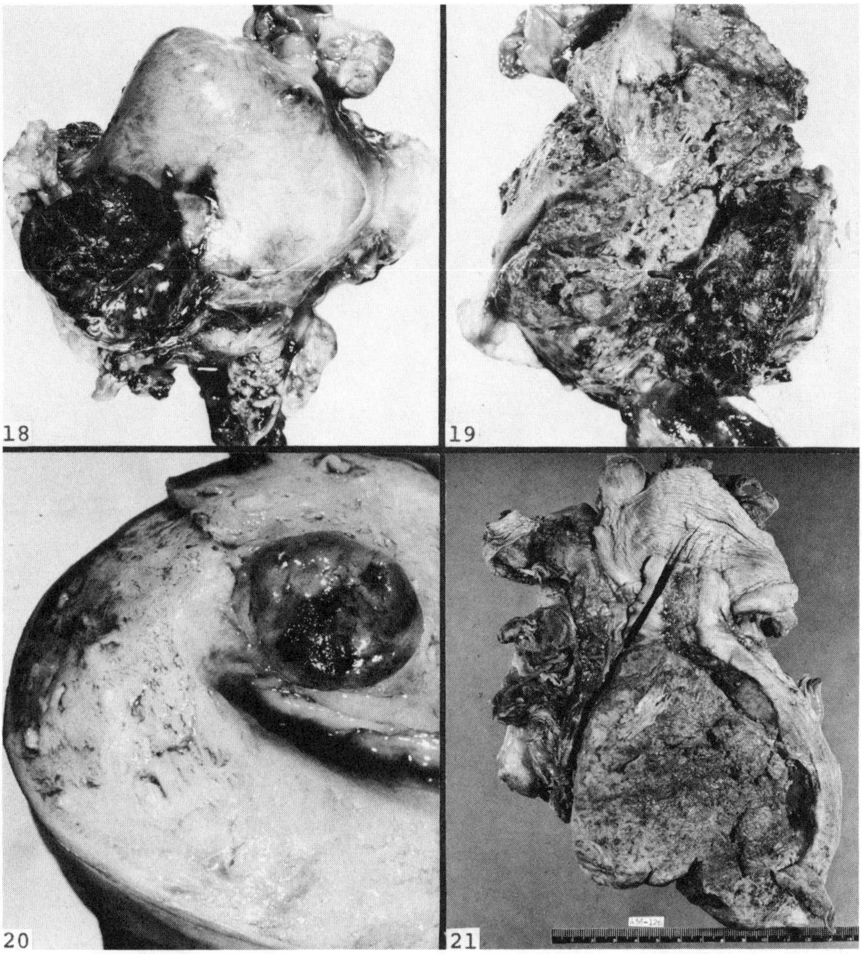

FIGURE 18. *Case 9:* Uterus at autopsy 8 months after term delivery and four courses of methotrexate and two of vincaleukoblastine. The fundus is perforated by choriocarcinoma giving rise to massive hemoperitoneum. Choriocarcinoma infiltrates the myometrium and right broad ligament. The ovaries are small, noncystic, and showed only minimal luteinization on microscopical examination.

FIGURE 19. *Case 9:* Uterus at autopsy, opened, showing the cavity filled with necrotic choriocarcinoma replacing the entire endometrium.

FIGURE 20. *Case 63:* Uterine fundus 3 months after term delivery, showing a spherical, apparently demarcated, focally hemorrhagic mass of choriocarcinoma in the myometrium impinging on the endometrial surface. Hysterectomy was performed prior to one course of methotrexate. Patient was reported living and well 10 years later.

FIGURE 21. *Case 23:* Pelvic contents at autopsy 15 months after a hydatidiform mole, showing destruction of the uterus by choriocarcinoma, which has also grown downward through the cervix and outward into the plevic soft tissue.

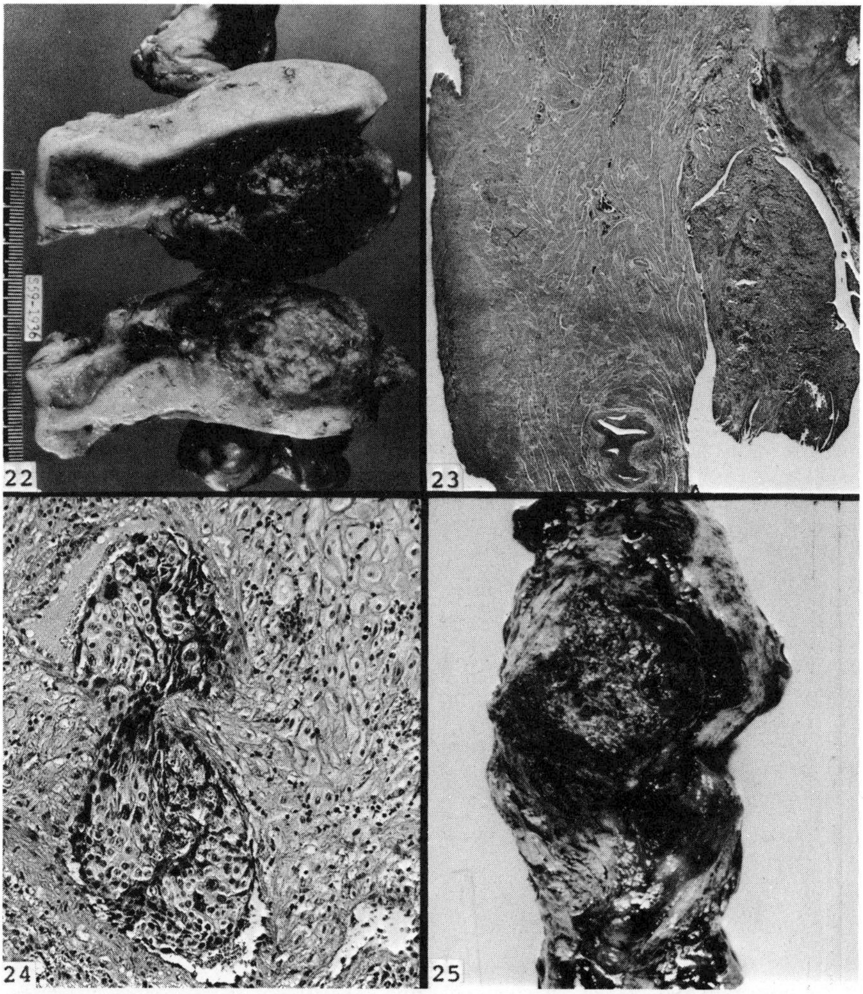

FIGURE 22. *Case 40:* Uterus, tubes, and ovaries removed 9 months after a spontaneous abortion, showing a large, friable, partly hemorrhagic mass infiltrating the fundus. Multiple small follicular cysts are seen in the ovarian cortices.

FIGURE 23. *Case 40:* Uterus 9 months after a spontaneous abortion, showing a superficial mass of choriocarcinoma with much hemorrhage. Permeation of the myometrium is not evident. (× 4)

FIGURE 24. *Case 40:* Uterine curettings 9 months after a spontaneous abortion, showing an embolus of choriocarcinoma in an endometrial venule. The surrounding stroma shows an intense decidual reaction. (× 104)

FIGURE 25. *Case 57:* Uterus at hysterectomy 1 year after term delivery, prior to chemotherapy, showing a large necrotic mass of choriocarcinoma projecting into the cavity and infiltrating the wall. Satellite nodules are scattered through the myometrium.

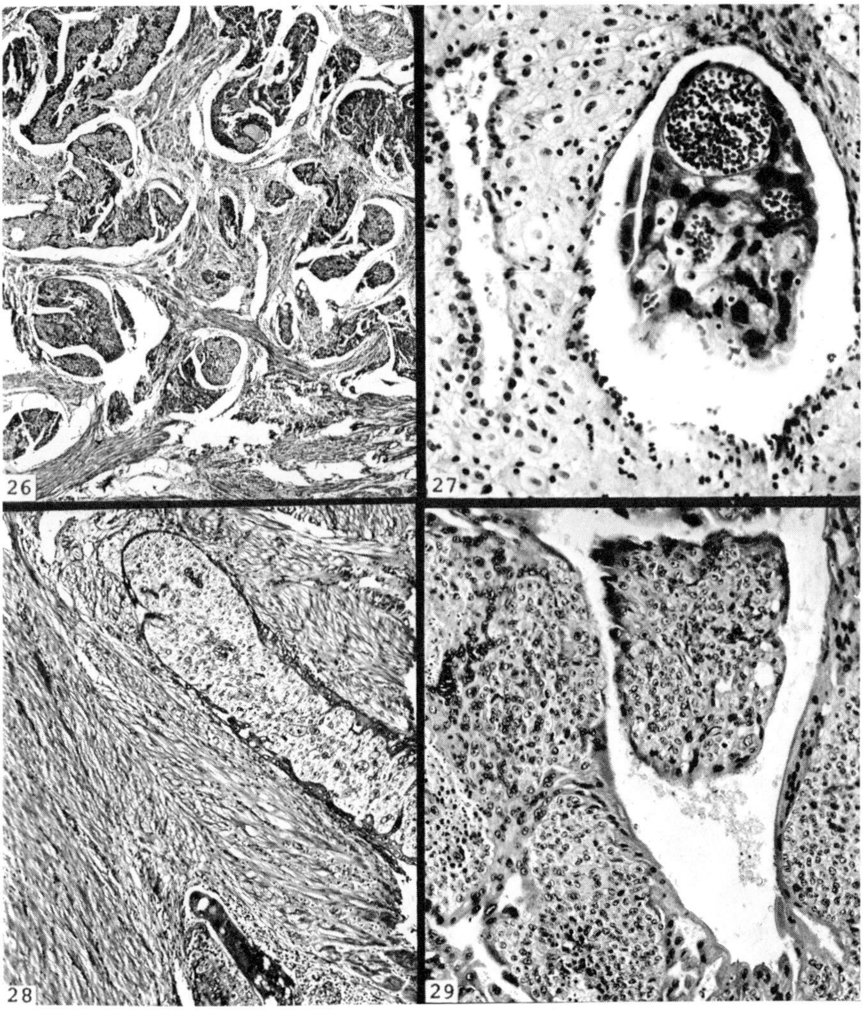

FIGURE 26. *Case 57:* Uterus showing diffuse, plexiform infiltration of the myometrium by choriocarcinoma. (× 14)

FIGURE 27. *Case 57:* Endometrial curettings 1 year after term delivery, showing an embolic fragment of choriocarcinoma in a dilated venule. The stroma shows an intense decidual reaction, and an endometrial gland shows exhaustion of secretory activity. (× 151)

FIGURE 28. *Case 57:* Uterus showing a tongue of choriocarcinoma infiltrating between smooth muscle bundles. A central core of cytotrophoblast with clear cytoplasm is surrounded by a sheath of attenuated syncytiotrophoblast with dark cytoplasm. (× 54)

FIGURE 29. *Case 57:* Endometrial curettings 1 year after term delivery, showing neoplastic trophoblast. (× 76)

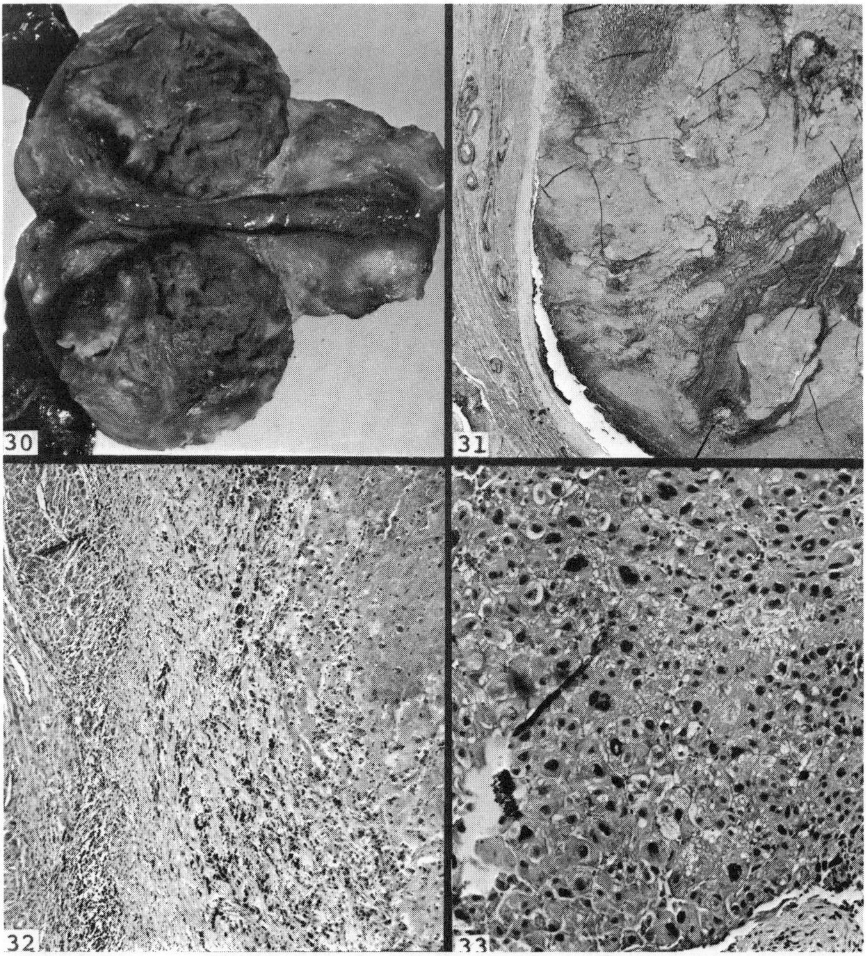

FIGURE 30. *Case 97:* Uterus, tubes, and ovaries removed 30 months after a hydatidiform mole and six courses of methotrexate. A necrotic spherical mass replaces three-fourths of the fundus; no viable tumor was found microscopically. The ovaries are small and free of cysts; 5 months previously, prior to hysterectomy, they had been greatly enlarged by theca-lutein cysts.

FIGURE 31. *Case 97:* Uterus at hysterectomy 30 months after a hyadtidiform mole and six courses of methotrexate, showing a portion of an entirely necrotic mass with no viable trophoblast. (× 5)

FIGURE 32. *Case 97:* Detail of FIGURE 31, showing zone of fibrosis and minimal lymphocytic reaction between the necrotic mass and the myometrium. (× 40)

FIGURE 33. *Case 84:* Uterine curettings 3 weeks after a hydatidiform mole, showing pleomorphic cytotrophoblast without chorionic villi. Hysterectomy 2 weeks later revealed invasive choriocarcinoma. (× 106)

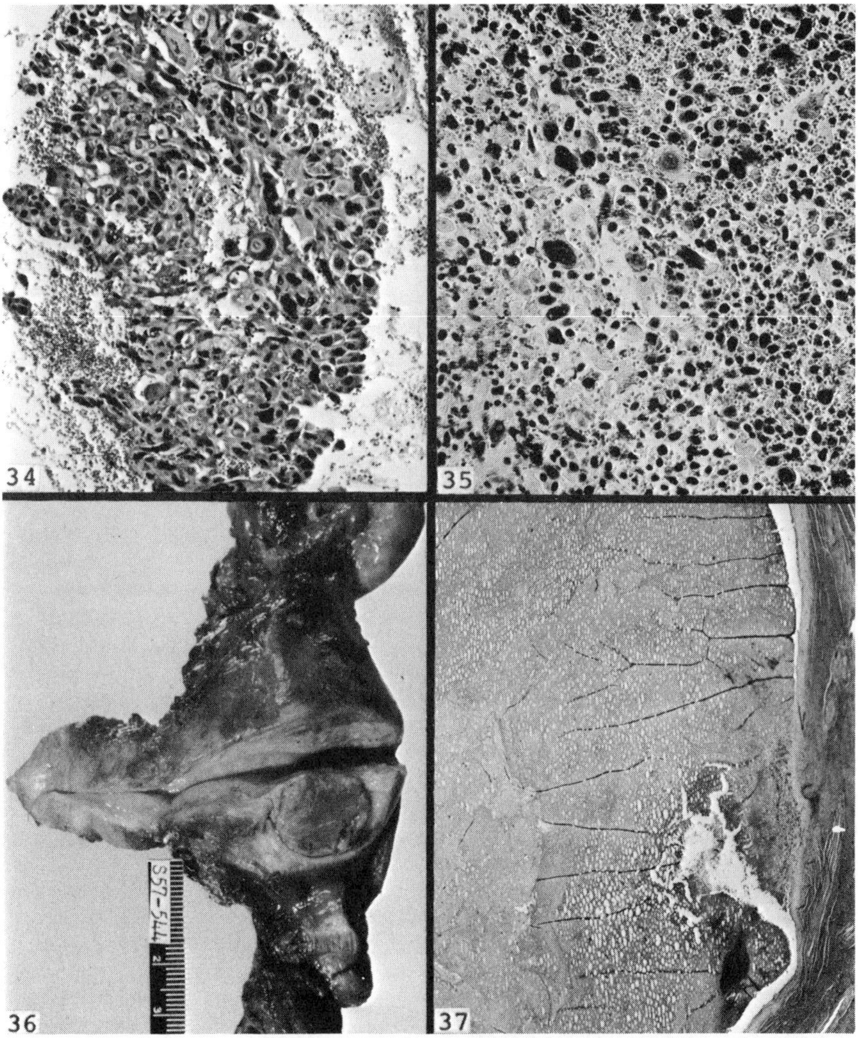

FIGURE 34. *Case 98:* Biopsy of a necrotic mass in a labium majust 19 months after term delivery, 44 months after a hydatidiform mole, showing atypical trophoblast without villi. (× 81)

FIGURE 35. *Case 98:* Detail of FIGURE 34, showing degenerating trophoblast with pyknotic, pleomorphic nuclei. (× 162) This case is classified as "probable" choriocarcinoma.

FIGURE 36. *Case 98:* Uterus, tubes, and ovaries 4 years and 8 months after a hydatidiform mole (see FIGURE 11); hysterectomy was performed after 17 courses of methotrexate. The myometrium contains a spherical necrotic mass 1.6 cm in diameter; no viable tumor was found microscopically. The ovaries were small and free from cysts or theca-lutein reaction.

FIGURE 37. *Case 98:* Uterus at hysterectomy 4 years and 8 months after a hydatidiform mole and 17 courses of methotrexate, showing a portion of the necrotic mass (see FIGURE 36) with no viable trophoblast. (× 40)

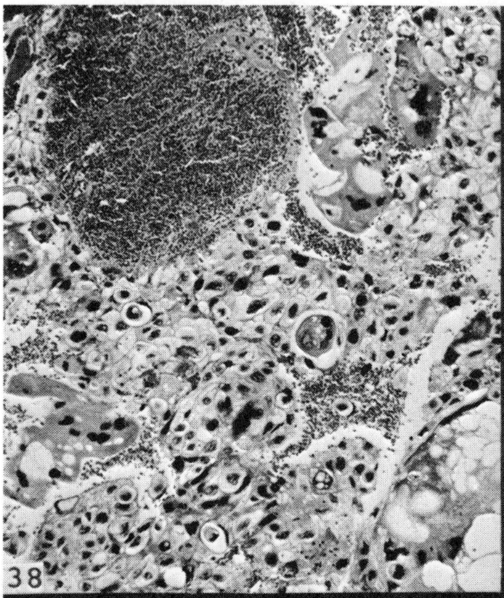

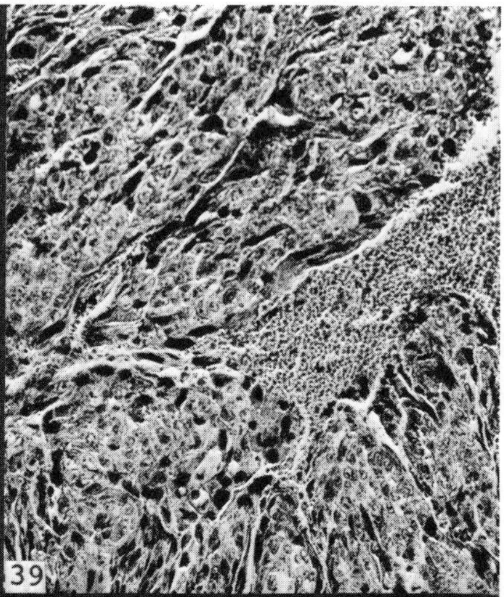

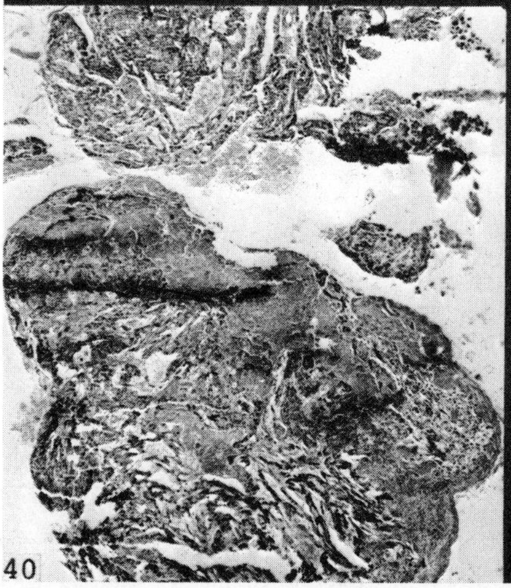

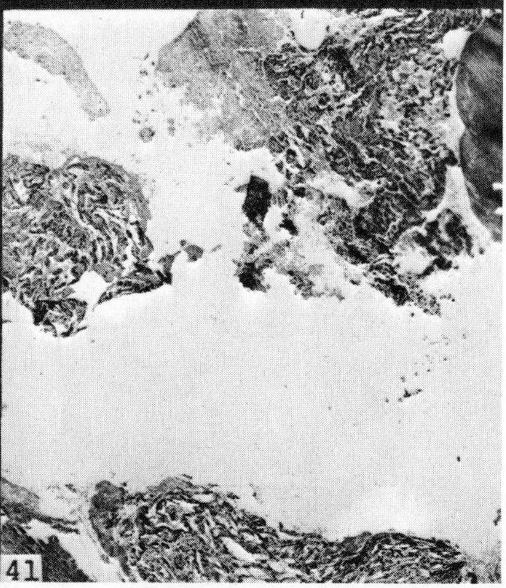

FIGURE 38. *Case 66:* Uterine curettings 5 weeks after delivery of an hydropic infant at 37 weeks of gestation. Disorderly proliferation of both cyto- and syncytiotrophoblast without villi warrants the diagnosis of choriocarcinoma. (× 57)

FIGURE 39. *Case 55:* Uterine curettings 6 weeks postpartum, showing typical choriocarcinoma containing both cyto- and syncytiotrophoblast. (× 115) Patient was reported well 5.5 years after delivery, following five courses of methotrexate.

FIGURE 40. *Case 64:* Uterine curettings 4 weeks postpartum. Despite histological inadequacies, the pattern of choriocarcinoma is unmistakable. (× 14)

FIGURE 41. *Case 64:* Another field from the same shown in FIGURE 40. (× 14)

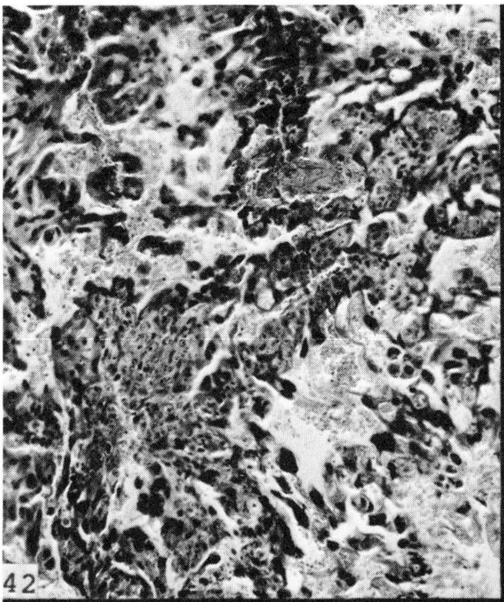

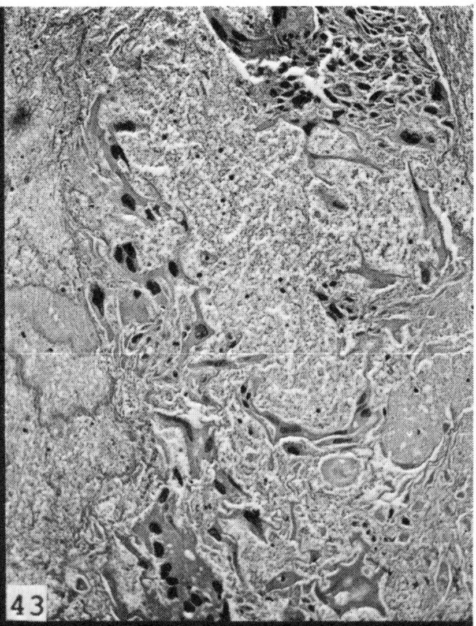

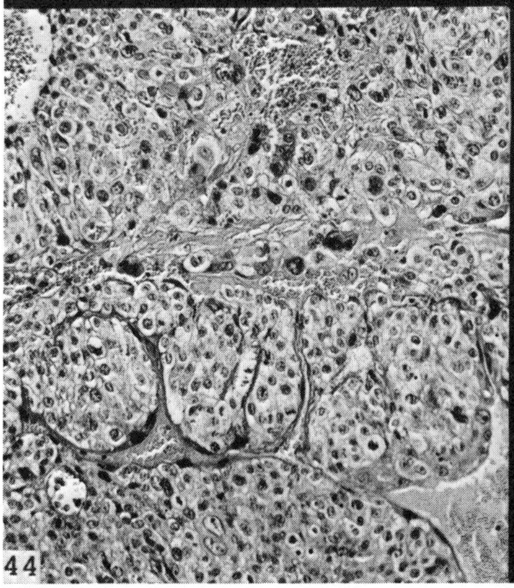

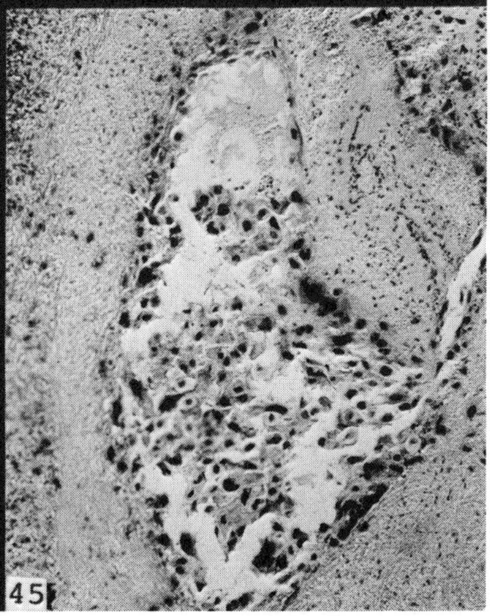

FIGURE 42. *Case 64:* Detail of FIGURE 40. (× 71) The patient received three courses of methotrexate, with remission. Normal pregnancy followed by cesarean section and hysterectomy 4 years after first delivery.

FIGURE 43. *Case 46:* Uterine curettings 4 weeks after term delivery, showing atypical trophoblast with extensive necrosis and degeneration. (× 85) Chest x-ray disclosed bilateral nodular densities in the lung fields. Patient had a partial remission with six courses of methotrexate and six courses of vincaleukoblastine, but died with clinical evidence of disseminated neoplasm 16 months after curettage; no autopsy was performed.

FIGURE 44. *Case 40:* Uterine curettings 2 months after a spontaneous abortion, showing masses of neoplastic trophoblast. (× 115)

FIGURE 45. *Case 88:* A single focus of atypical trophoblastic proliferation in curettings for spontaneous incomplete abortion. Hysterectomy 13 months later showed invasive choriocarcinoma. (× 81)

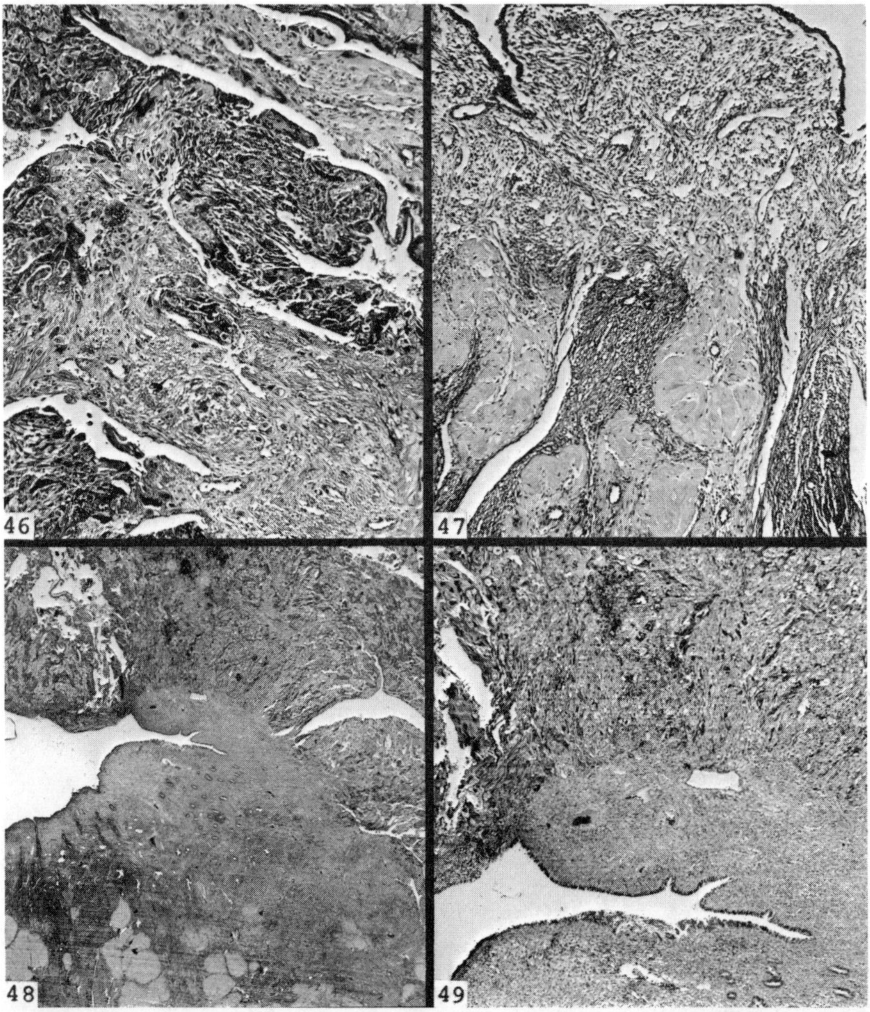

FIGURE 46. *Case 59:* Uterus at hysterectomy 2 months postpartum, showing choriocarcinoma infiltrating the myometrium. (× 48)

FIGURE 47. *Case 59:* Area 3–4 mm away from that shown in FIGURE 46, showing placental site with partially regenerated endometrium, and involuted vessesls with hyaline collars, but no choriocarcinoma. (× 48) Patient received one course of nitrogen mustard after hysterectomy and was free of disease when admitted to NIH; this is essentially an untreated case, with an 11-year survival following hysterectomy.

FIGURE 48. *Case 67:* Uterus at hysterectomy 10 weeks postpartum, showing a polypoid extrusion of a largely exophytic choriocarcinoma adjacent to the placental site and covered by regenerated endometrium. (× 10)

FIGURE 49. *Case 67:* Detail of FIGURE 48, showing choriocarcinoma underlying the regenerated endometrium. (× 21)

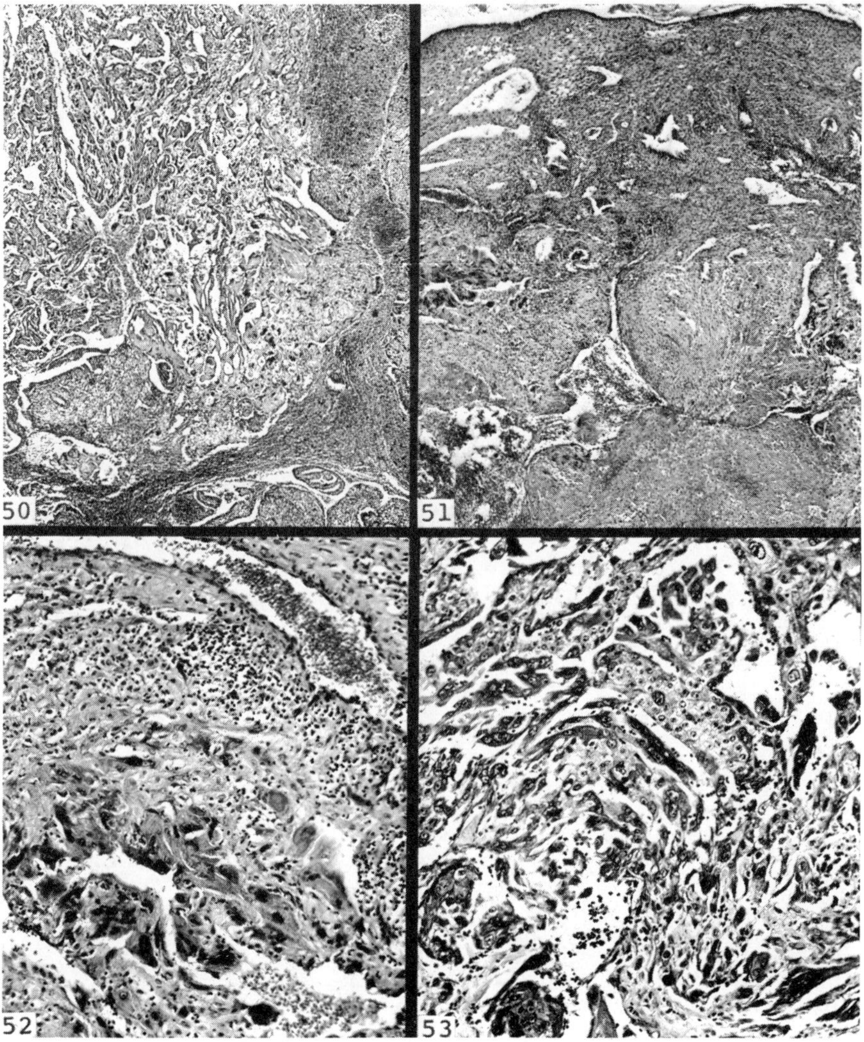

FIGURE 50. *Case 67:* Detail of FIGURE 48, showing pattern of neoplastic trophoblast. (× 26)

FIGURE 51. *Case 25:* Uterine curettings 18 months after a hydatidiform mole, showing regenerated endomertium with persistent decdiual reaction and dilated venules. A few clusters of trophoblastic cells with hyperchromatic nuclei are present, as well as a zone of necrosis. (× 32)

FIGURE 52. *Case 25:* Detail of FIGURE 51, showing the bizarre trophoblast diagnosed as "suspicious for choriocarcinoma." (× 92)

FIGURE 53. *Case 47:* Uterus at hysterectomy 5 months after curettage for incomplete spontaneous abortion, showing infiltrating choriocarcinoma. (× 92)

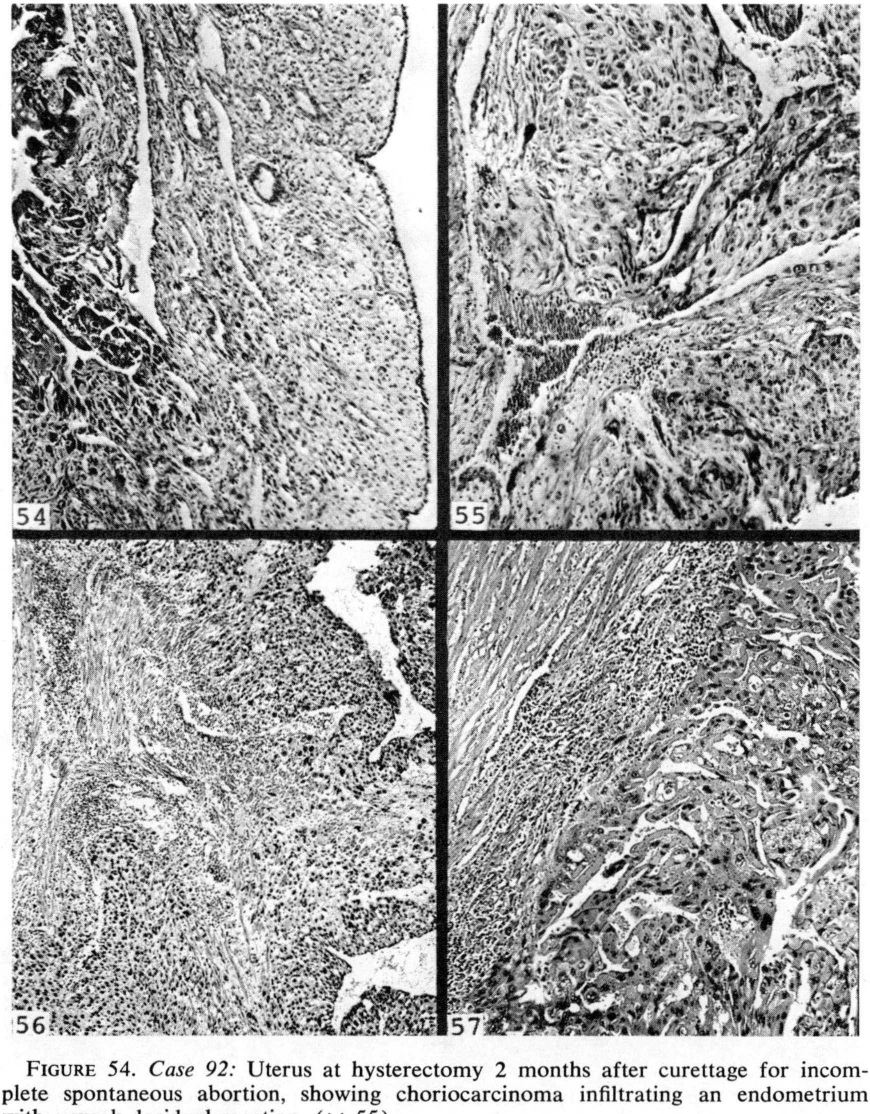

FIGURE 54. *Case 92:* Uterus at hysterectomy 2 months after curettage for incomplete spontaneous abortion, showing choriocarcinoma infiltrating an endometrium with a weak decidual reaction. (× 55)

FIGURE 55. *Case 92:* View of a deeper portion of the tumor shown in FIGURE 54, showing choriocarcinoma invading the myometrium and a uterine vein. (× 71)

FIGURE 56. *Case 38:* Uterus 10 weeks after a spontaneous abortion, showing choriocarcinoma invading the myometrium. A moderately prominent zone of lymphocytic reaction lies between the advancing tumor margin and the uterine smooth muscle. (× 37)

FIGURE 57. *Case 93:* Uterus at hysterectomy 2 months after a spontaneous incomplete abortion, showing a narrow zone of lymphocytic infiltration between the advancing choriocarcinoma and the myometrium. (× 55)

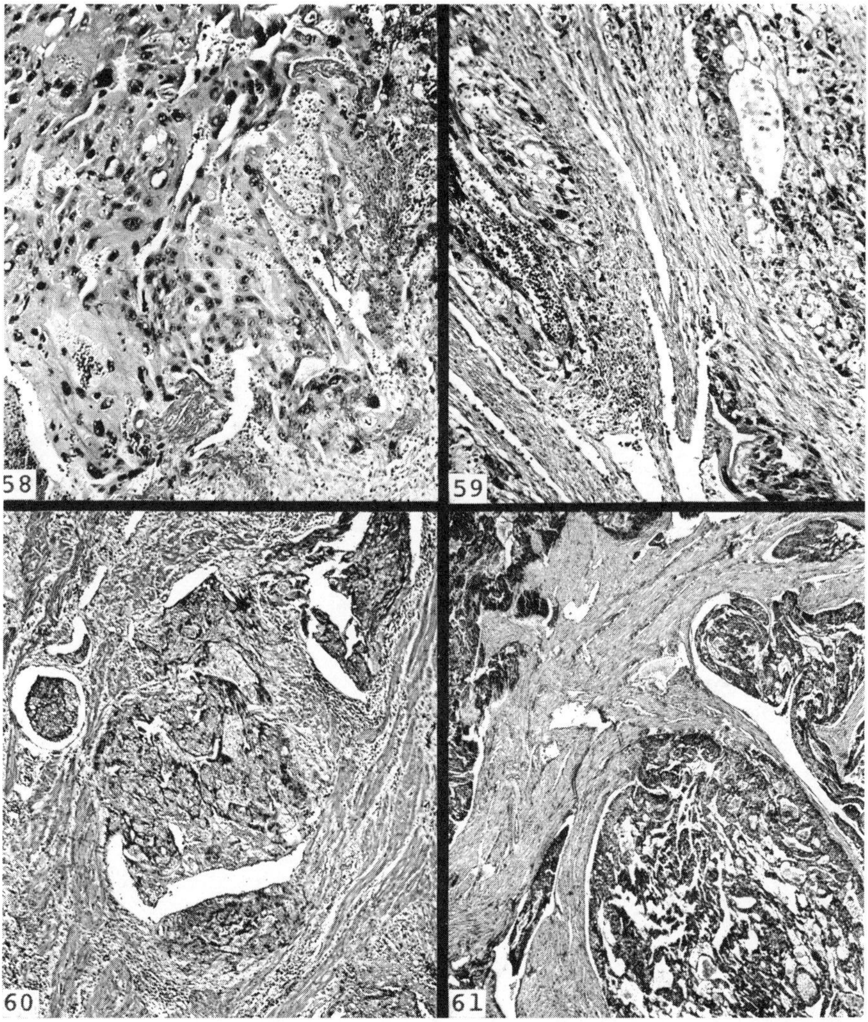

FIGURE 58. *Case 56:* Uterus at hysterectomy 3 months postpartum, showing choriocarcinoma infiltrating the myometrium. (× 60) Patient had a 13-year survival after eight courses of methotrexate.

FIGURE 59. *Case 5:* Uterus at hysterectomy 5 weeks postpartum, showing diffuse infiltration by choriocarcinoma. (× 92)

FIGURE 60. *Case 89:* Uterus at hysterectomy 6 months after curettage for incomplete spontaneous abortion, showing invasion of the myometrium and myometrial veins by choriocarcinoma. Thin zones of lymphocytic reaction abut the neoplastic infiltration. (× 39)

FIGURE 61. *Case 84:* Uterus at hysterectomy 1 month after a hydatidiform mole (see FIGURE 7), showing large masses of choriocarcinoma invading the myometrium and myometrial veins. (× 26)

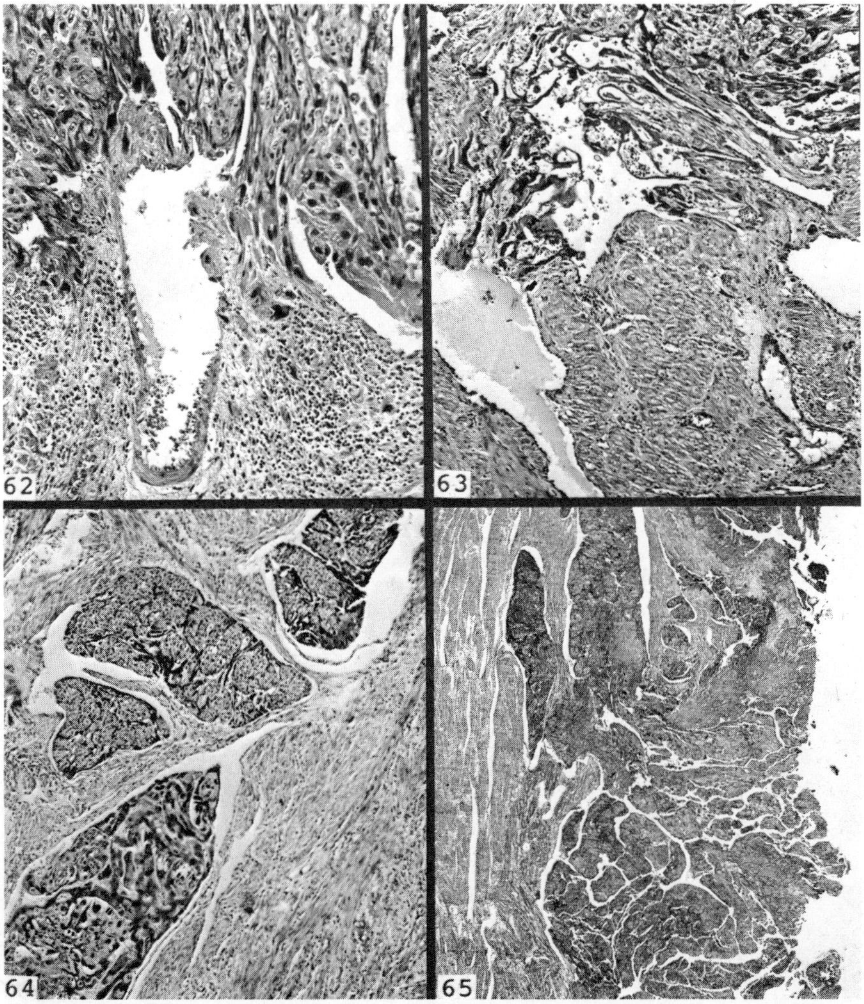

FIGURE 62. *Case 60:* Uterus at hysterectomy 11 weeks after term delivery, showing a segment of the edge of infiltrating choriocarcinoma. An open myometrial vein is being entered by advancing neoplasm. (× 85)

FIGURE 63. *Case 7:* Uterus at hysterectomy 7 weeks postpartum, showing choriocarcinoma invading a dilated vein in the myometrium. (× 55)

FIGURE 64. *Case 90:* Uterus at hysterectomy 15 weeks after criminal abortion, showing invasion of the myometrial veins by choriocarcinoma. (× 43)

FIGURE 65. *Case 76:* Uterus at hysterectomy 4 months after a hydatidiform mole was evacuated by hysterotomy. The endometrium is replaced by infiltrating choriocarcinoma. (× 11)

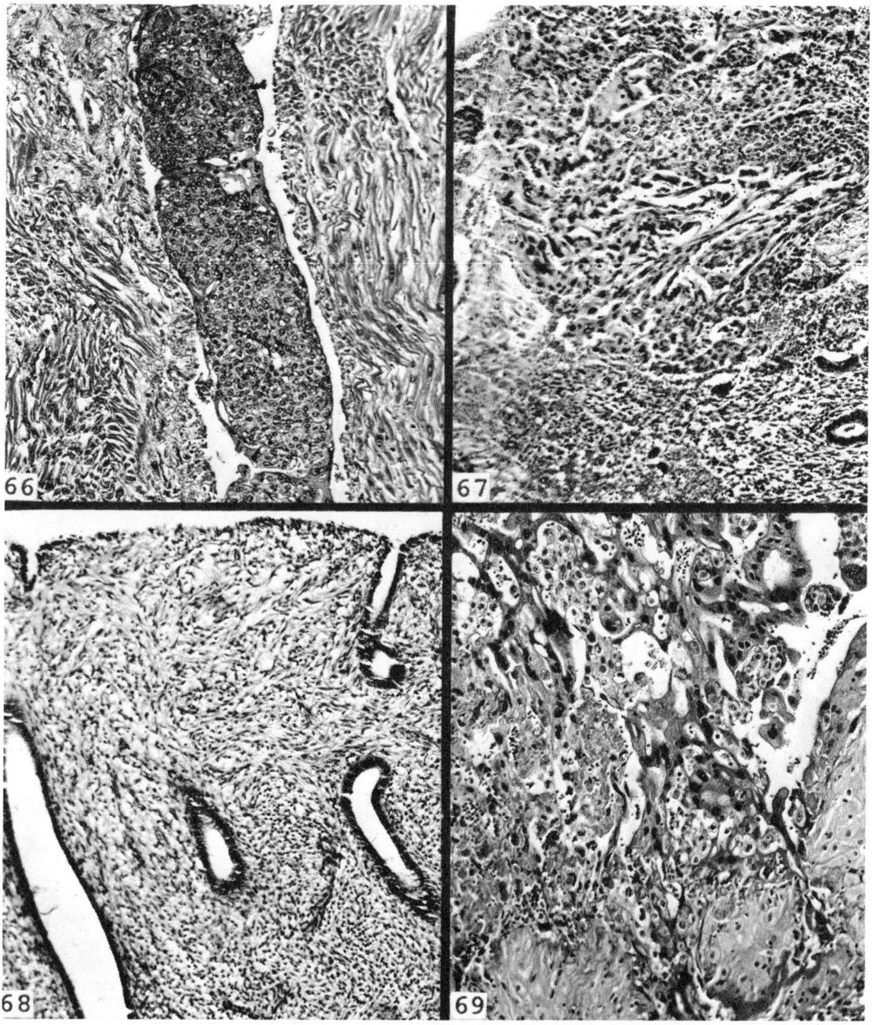

FIGURE 66. *Case 76:* Detail of FIGURE 65, showing a tongue of choriocarcinoma infiltrating the myometrium. The central core of cytotrophoblast is covered by an attenuated layer of syncytiotrophoblast, and a few lymphocytes are sprinkled in the nearby myometrium. (× 106)

FIGURE 67. *Case 19:* Endometrium at hysterectomy 3 months after a hydatidiform mole, showing invasive choriocarcinoma. (× 77)

FIGURE 68. *Case 19:* Endometrium near that shown in FIGURE 67 is composed of tubular glands without secretion or mitoses, a stroma without decidua-like reaction, and undeveloped spiral arterioles. (× 64)

FIGURE 69. *Case 25:* Uterus at hysterectomy 19 months after a hydatidiform mole, showing choriocarcinoma (see FIGURES 51 and 52). (× 102)

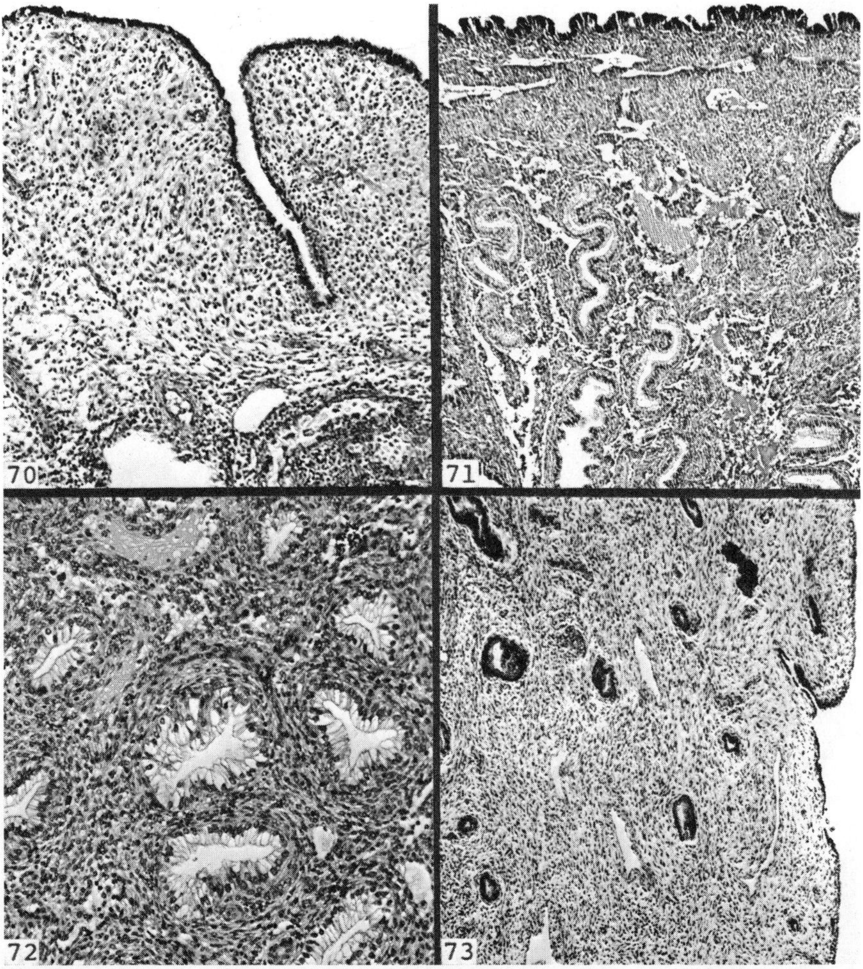

FIGURE 70. *Case 25:* Endometrium showing a weak decidua-like reaction. A gland in the stratum basalis shows an Arias-Stella reaction. (× 71)

FIGURE 71. *Case 63:* Endometrium at hysterectomy 3 months after term delivery, showing early secretory phase with no decidual reaction in the stroma. Elsewhere, the uterus was infiltrated by choriocarcinoma. The ovaries were not removed. (× 51)

FIGURE 72. *Case 84:* Endometrium at hysterectomy 1 month after a hydatidiform mole, showing convoluted glands with supranuclear secretory vacuoles and a cellular stroma without predecidual reaction. A Friedman test was positive at 1:1,000 dilution (see FIGURES 7 and 61). (× 106)

FIGURE 73. *Case 1:* Endometrium at autopsy 1 year after term delivery, showing slightly coiled glands without mitoses or secretion and a weak decidua-like reaction in the stroma. No choriocarcinoma was found in the uterus itself. The terminal HCG titer was approximately 100,000 units. (× 47)

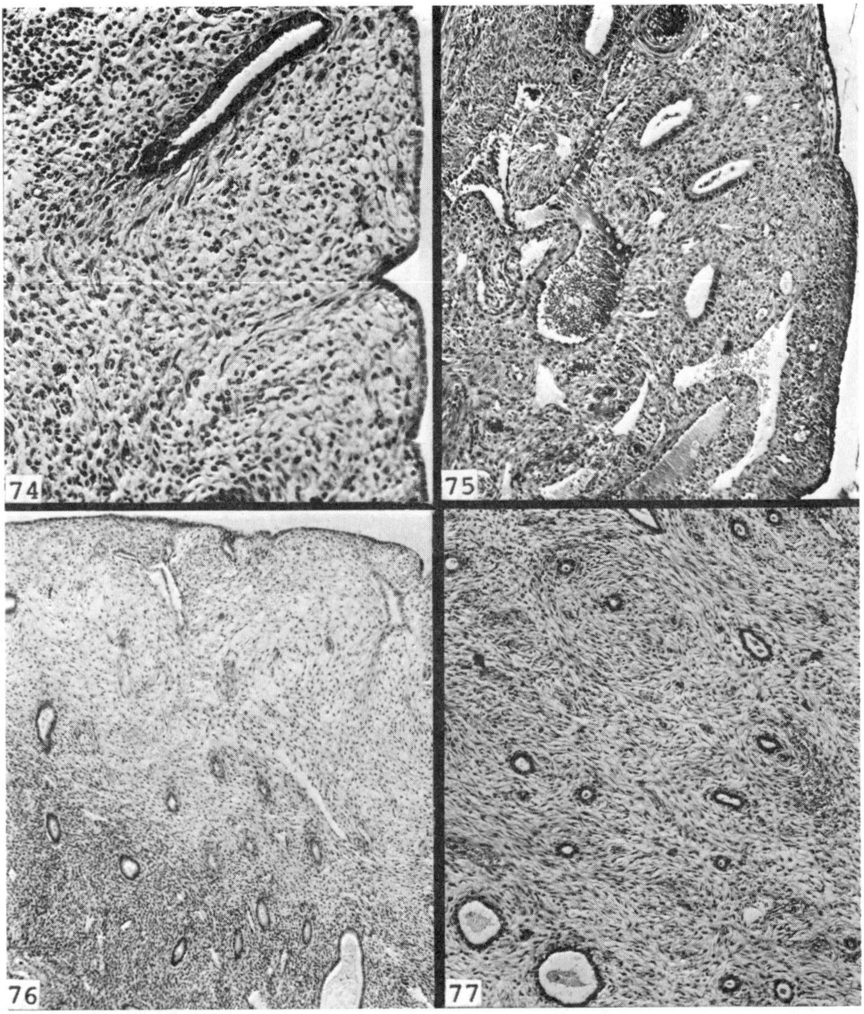

FIGURE 74. *Case 1:* Detail of FIGURE 73, at higher magnification. (× 128)

FIGURE 75. *Case 57:* Endometrium 11 months after term delivery, showing a rather thin mucosa composed of glands with exhausted secretion, a decidua-like stroma, and dilated venules. Spiral arterioles are not well developed. Choriocarcinoma was found in curettings 1 month later (see FIGURES 25–29). (× 64)

FIGURE 76. *Case 15:* Endometrium at autopsy 1 year after term delivery, showing glands of small caliber lined by cuboidal epithelium without mitoses or secretion. The stroma is lose, with superficial edema, and free of predecidual reaction. Spiral arterioles are not developed. HCG titer was >200,000 units. The pattern resembles that produced by synthetic estrogen-progestagen preparations. (× 26)

FIGURE 77. *Case 15:* Deeper layers of the endometrium shown in FIGURE 76, at higher magnification. (× 55)

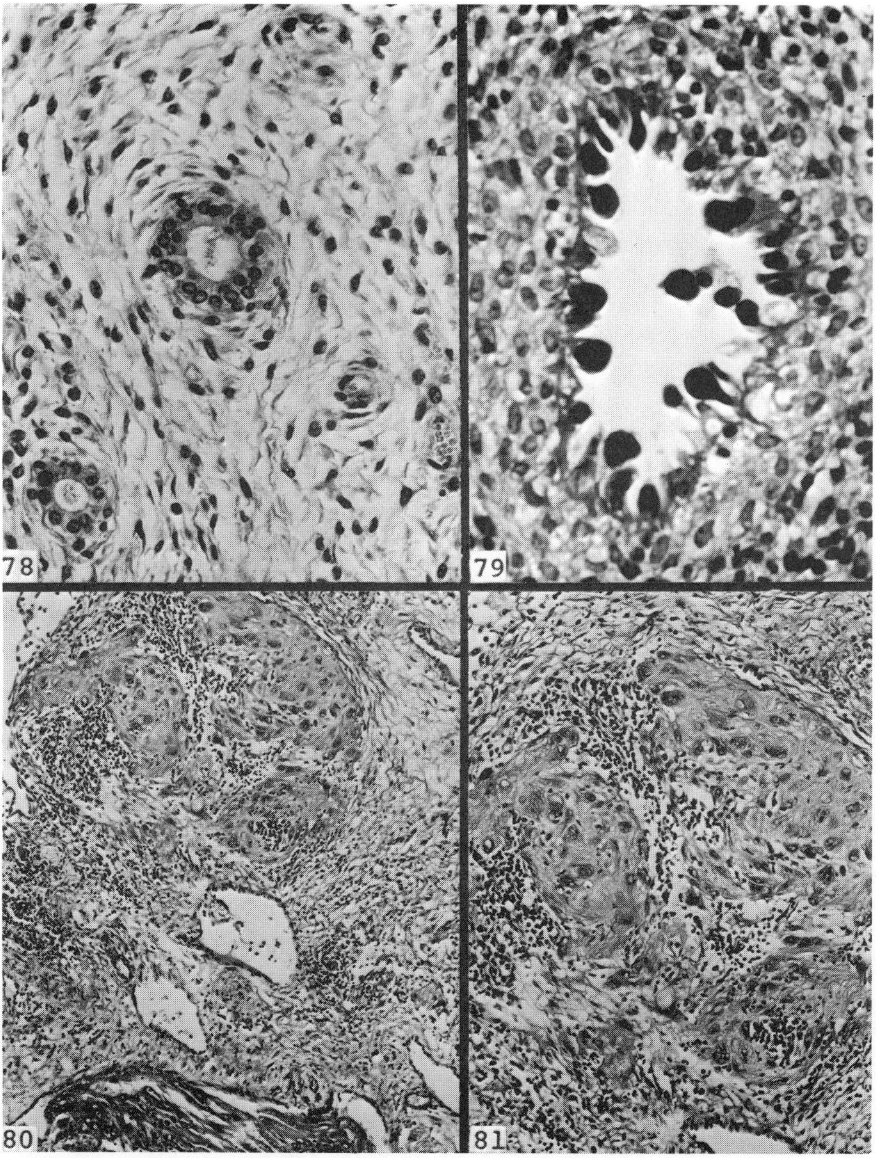

FIGURE 78. *Case 15:* Detail of FIGURE 77, at higher magnification. (× 189)

FIGURE 79. *Case 31:* Uterine curettings 12 weeks after a hydatidiform mole, showing an unsual Arias-Stella effect in an endometrial gland. (× 122)

FIGURE 80. *Case 12:* Parametrial tissue 8 months postpartum, showing infiltration by choriocarcinoma extending directly from uterus. Parametrial veins are dilated, and there is an ectopic decidual reaction in the soft tissue. (× 63)

FIGURE 81. *Case 12:* Detail of FIGURE 80, showing ectopic decidua. (× 108)

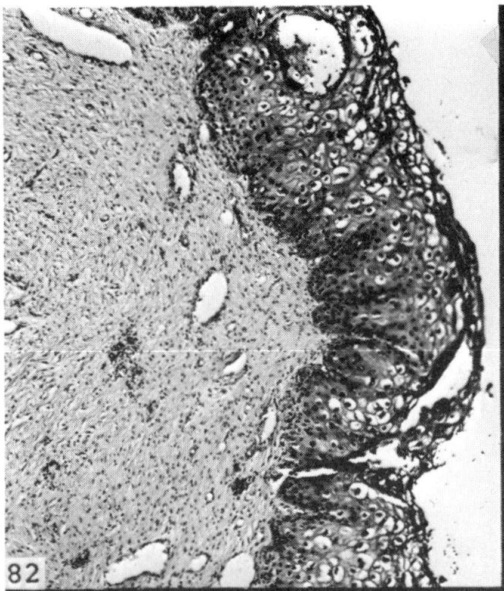

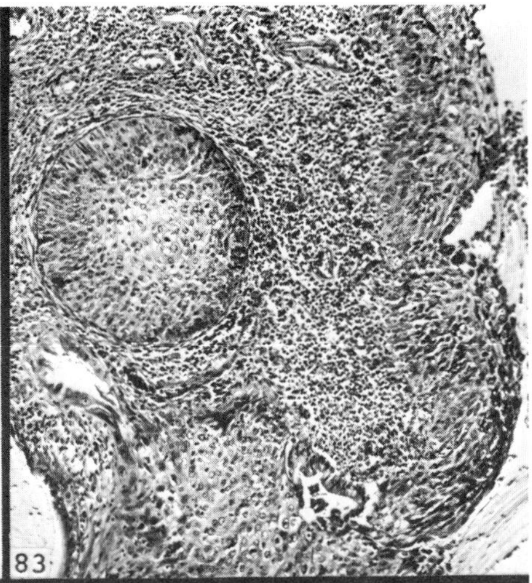

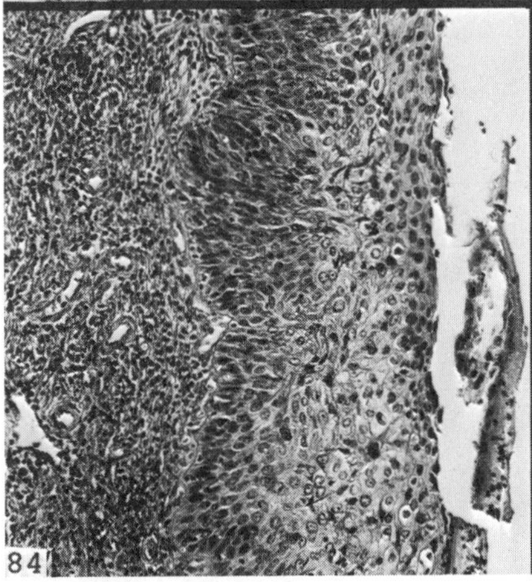

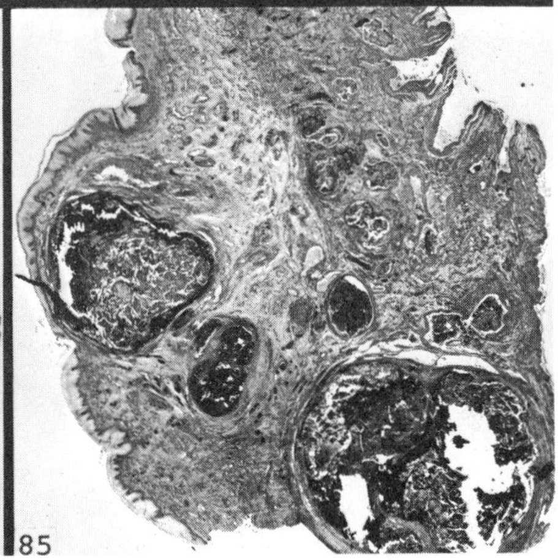

FIGURE 82. *Case 80:* Exocervix at hysterectomy 8.5 years after a hydatidiform mole. The Friedman test was positive, but the uterus contained no tumor. The focus of squamous cells with pyknotic nuclei surrounded by clear perinuclear cytoplasm resembles an effect sometimes seen in normal pregnancy. A nodule of metastatic choriocarcinoma was removed at pulmonary lobectomy 3 months later. (× 45)

FIGURE 83. *Case 39:* Cervix at autopsy 14 months after a spontaneous abortion, showing dysplastic squamous epithelium covering the endocervical surface and extending into endocervical glands. A portion of one gland dilated by inspissated excess mucus secretion is shown, resembling an effect seen in normal pregnancy. (× 68)

FIGURE 84. *Case 25:* Exocervix at hysterectomy 19 months after a hydatidiform mole. The uterus contained choriocarcinoma. The squamous epithelium shows moderate dysplastic changes, with hyperplasia of the basal cell layer and some disarray of cells in the stratum spinosum. (× 120)

FIGURE 85. *Case 4:* Vagina at autopsy 8 months after term delivery, showing permeation of the submucosal veins by masses of embolic neoplastic trophoblast. Essentially an untreated case. (× 5.6)

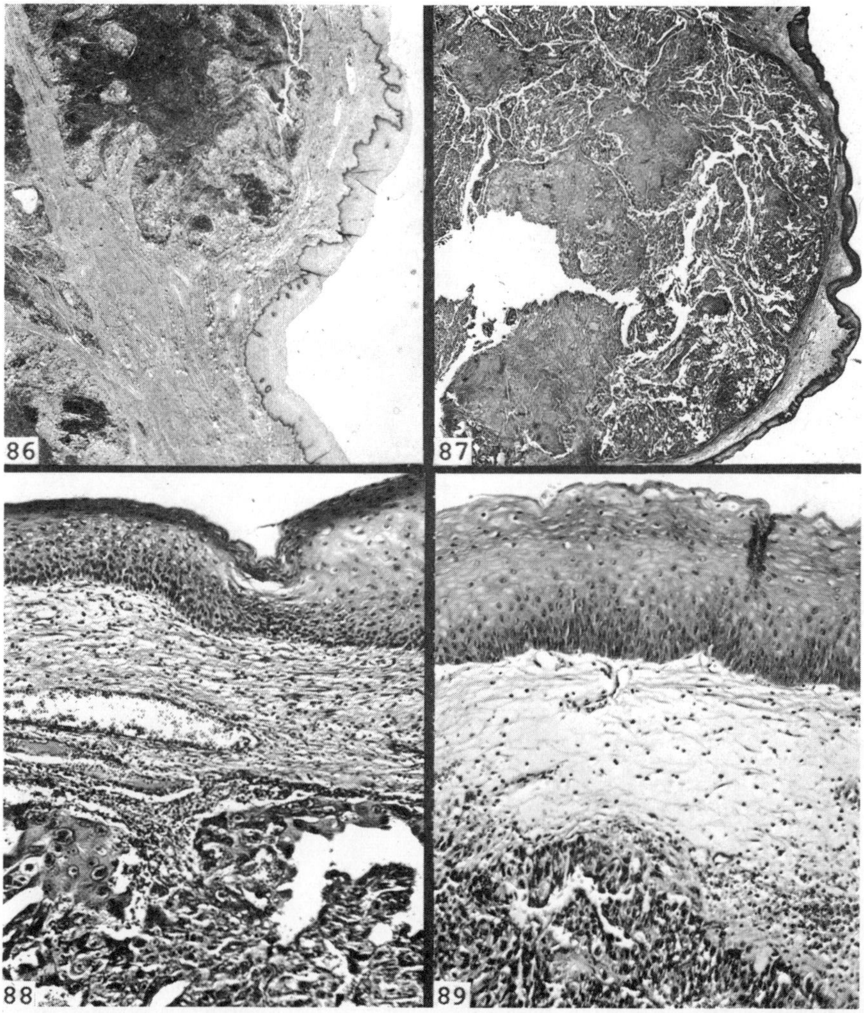

FIGURE 86. *Case 5:* Vagina at autopsy 7 months after term delivery, showing diffuse infiltration by metastatic choriocarcinoma. The vaginal mucosa was ulcerated, and there is hemorrhage within the tumor (see FIGURE 59). (× 10)

FIGURE 87. *Case 57:* Vaginal nodule 1 year after term delivery, showing the submucosa replaced by a large mass of trophoblast with central hemorrhage. The mucosa is thinned at the apex of the nodule, and ulceration seems imminent (see FIGURES 25–29). (× 6)

FIGURE 88. *Case 57:* Detail of FIGURE 87, showing sheets of cytotrophoblast and syncytiotrophoblast forming pseudovascular spaces. A dilated venule lies between the tumor and the vaginal mucosa. (× 85)

FIGURE 89. *Case 91:* Vaginal nodule 9 months after abortion, showing sheets of trophoblast infiltrating the submucosa. (× 92)

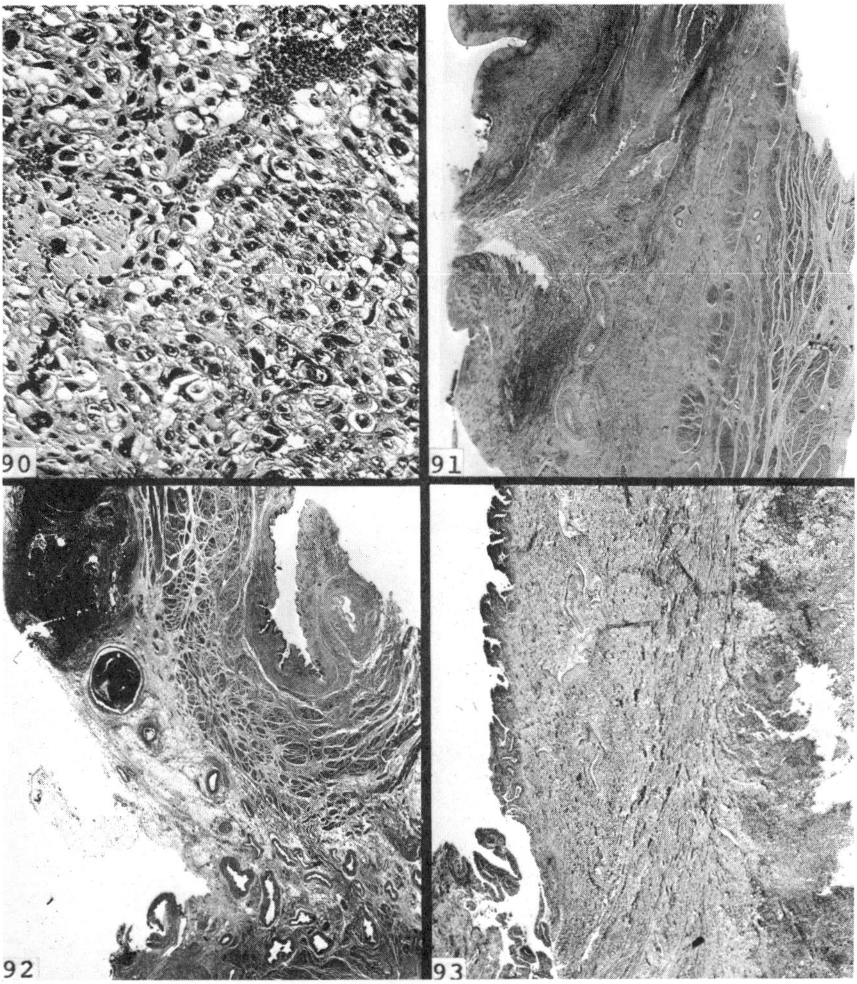

FIGURE 90. *Case 91:* Tissue deep to that shown in FIGURE 89, showing sheetlike growth and pleomorphism of trophoblast. (× 115)

FIGURE 91. *Case 16:* Vagina at autopsy 23 months after term delivery, showing a zone of necrosis, fibrosis, and hemosiderin phagocytosis consistent with a healed secondary deposit of choriocarcinoma. The patient had received five courses of methotrexate and five of actinomycin-D, but died of hemorrhage from a cerebral metastasis despite healing of secondary deposits in the lungs and vagina. (× 4)

FIGURE 92. *Case 9:* Bladder, vesicovaginal septum, and anterior vaginal wall 8 months postpartum, showing a hemorrhagic nodule of choriocarcinoma deposited on the dome of the bladder. An adjacent vein is thrombosed. (× 4)

FIGURE 93. *Case 5:* Bladder at autopsy 7 months postpartum, showing diffuse infiltration by choriocarcinoma. The tumor had ulcerated through the mucosa and showed extensive necrosis (see FIGURES 59 & 86.) (× 14)

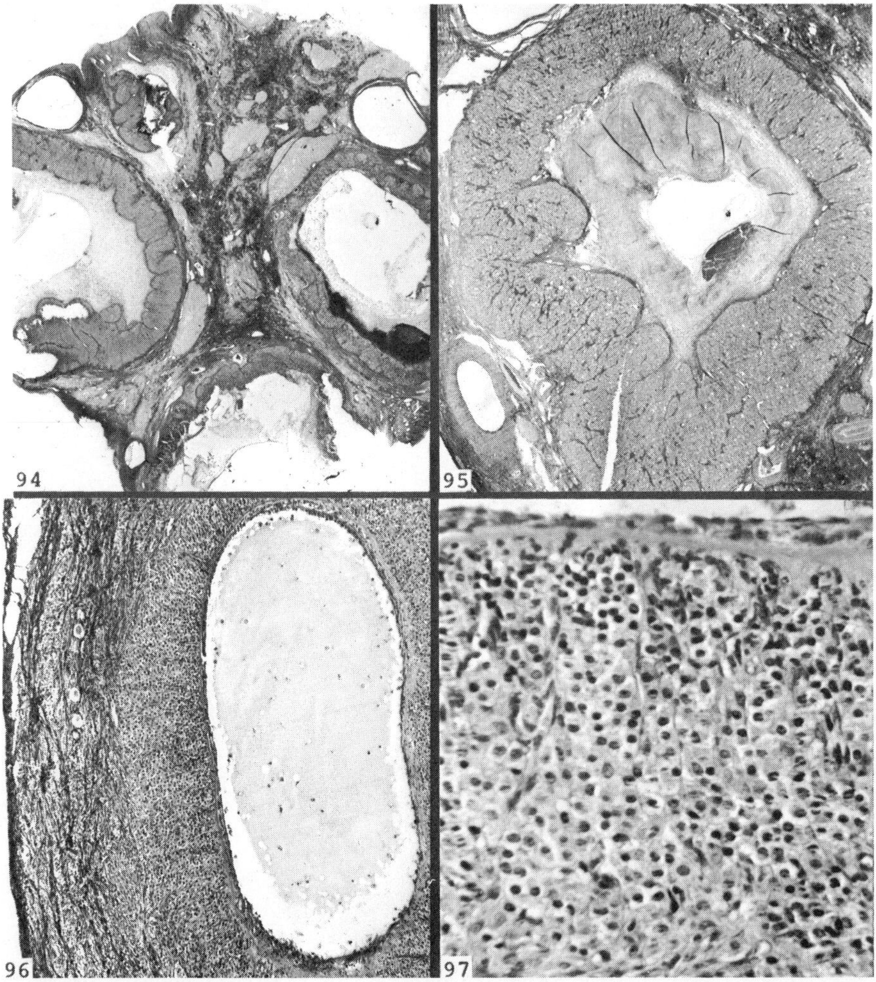

FIGURE 94. *Case 82:* Ovary at laparotomy 2 months after a hydatidiform mole, showing multiple luteinized cysts as well as a persistent corpus luteum gestations. The HCG titer was 25,000 units at the time. (× 3)

FIGURE 95. *Case 30:* Ovary 6 months after a hydatidiform mole, showing a well-formed corpus luteum with a small theca-lutein cyst between it and the surface. The HCG titer was 200,000 units. (× 8)

FIGURE 96. *Case 30:* Detail of FIGURE 95, showing the small theca-lutein cyst in the ovarian cortex. (× 43)

FIGURE 97. *Case 30:* Detail of FIGURE 96, showing the luteinized theca cells. (× 198)

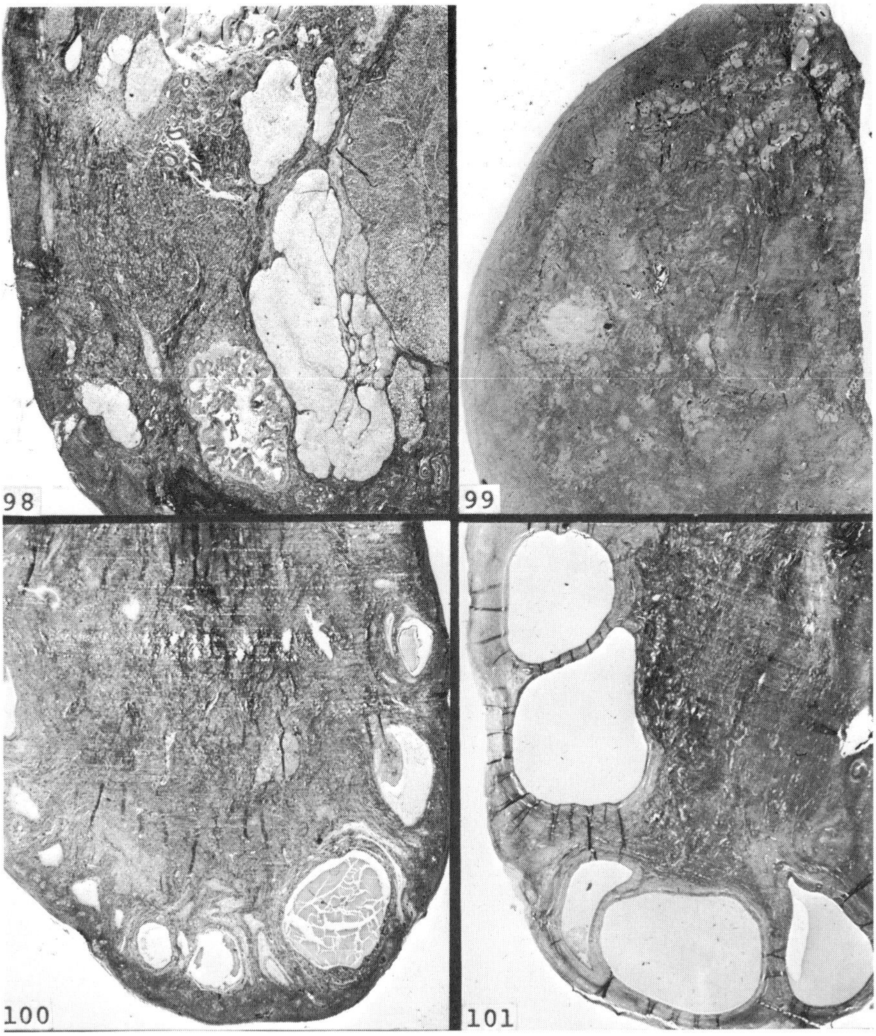

FIGURE 98. *Case 20:* Ovary at autopsy 23 months after a hydatidiform mole, showing a persistent corpus luteum, marked stromal luteinization, and ectopic decidual plaques. (× 7)

FIGURE 99. *Case 35:* Ovary at autopsy 23 months after a hydatidiform mole. There are no cysts and no evidence of luteinization; a few corpora albicantia are present in the medulla. The terminal HCG titer was >500,000 units. (× 2.6)

FIGURE 100. *Case 43:* Ovary at autopsy 1 month after choriocarcinoma was diagnosed at craniotomy. Cystically expanded follicles surrounded by mantles of theca interna are lined up beneath the tunica albuginea. The theca is minimally luteinized. The medullary stroma is hypercellular. Small patches of ectopic decidua are present. (× 4)

FIGURE 101. *Case 66:* Ovary at laparotomy 11 weeks postpartum, showing multiple cystic follicles lined up beneath a slightly thickened tunica albuginea. The cystic follicles are surrounded by prominent mantles of theca interna. An old corpus albicans and the regressing corpus luteum gestationis are seen in the medulla (see FIGURE 38). (× 6)

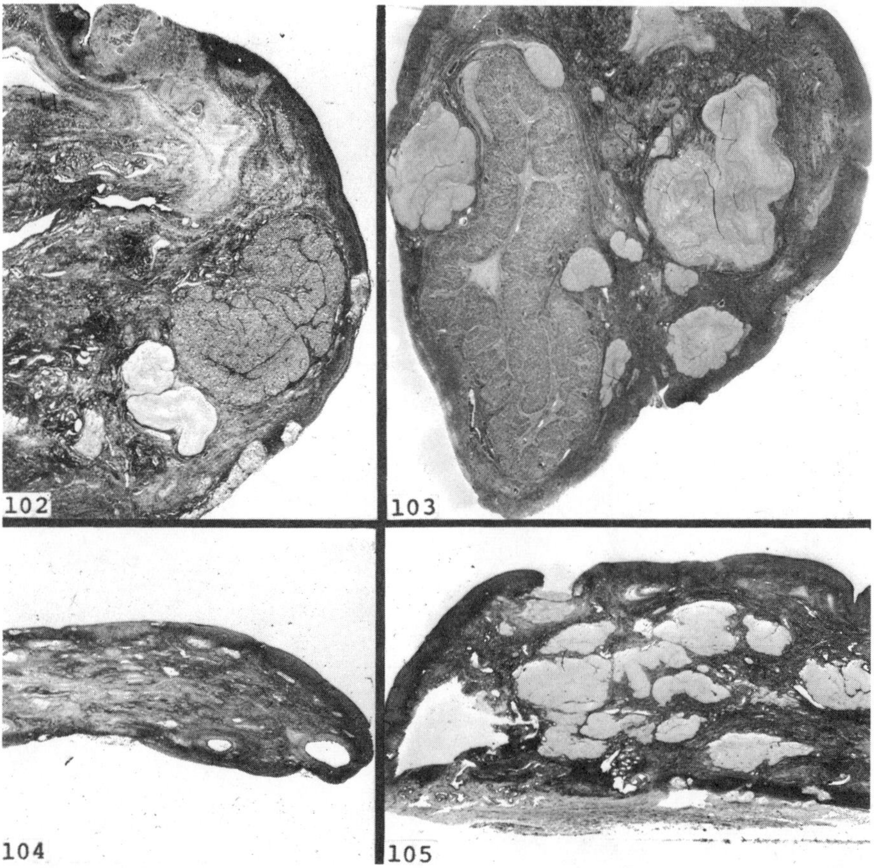

FIGURE 102. *Case 3:* Ovary at autopsy 10 months postpartum, showing plaques of ectopic decidua, a regressing corpus luteum, and slight stromal luteinization. (× 5)

FIGURE 103. *Case 11:* Ovary at autopsy 10 months after term delivery. A corpus luteum is present, as are few tiny plaques of ectopic decidua, but there are no cysts, no theca-lutein reaction, and no stromal luteinization. The ovary resembles a normal ovary in an ovulating woman. (× 4)

FIGURE 104. *Case 1:* Ovary at autopsy 1 year postpartum, showing moderate atrophy of both cortex and medulla. Three small cysts lined by weakly luteinized theca cells are present. Hypophysectomy was performed 6 weeks before death, but the terminal HCG titer was >50,000 units. × 3)

FIGURE 105. *Case 15:* Ovary at autopsy 12 months after term delivery, showing normal corticomedullary proportions, no cysts, many corpora albicantia in the medulla, and small plaques of ectopic decidua at the cortical surface. (× 3)

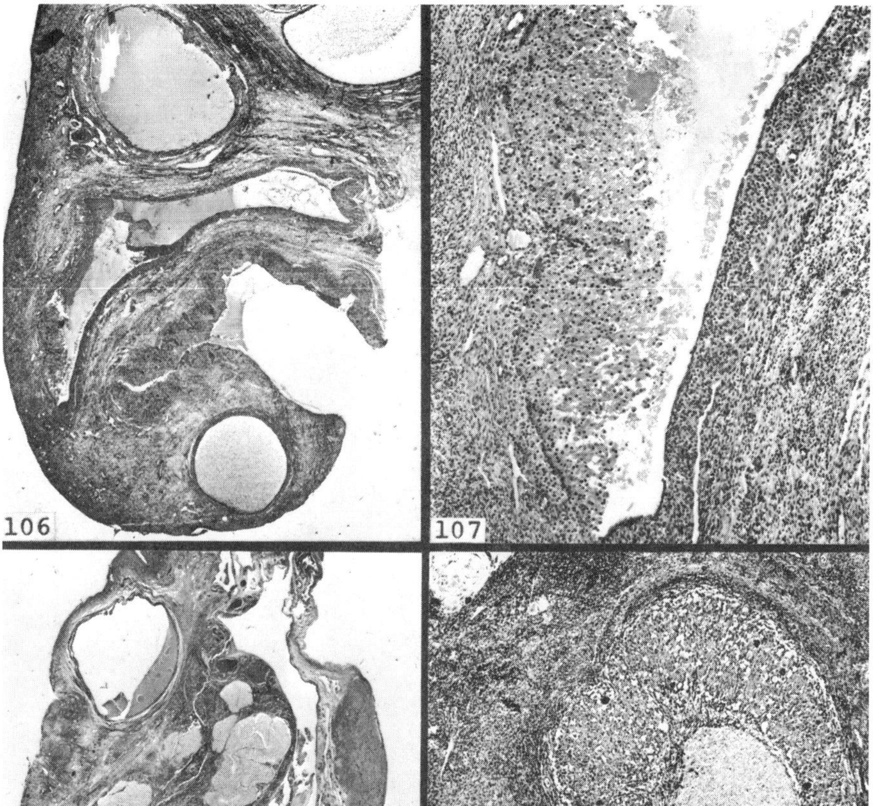

FIGURE 106. *Case 57:* Ovary at laparotomy 1 year postpartum, showing multiple theca-lutein cysts. The uterus was diffusely infiltrated by choriocarcinoma. (× 9)

FIGURE 107. *Case 57:* Detail of FIGURE 106, showing luteinized theca cells and a patch of luteinized granulosa cells. (× 49)

FIGURE 108. *Case 41:* Ovary at laparotomy 15 weeks after a spontaneous abortion. The uterus contained choriocarcinoma. The ovarian cortex is of normal thickness, and the medulla contains many corpora albicantia. A single cystic follicle is seen, and there is no luteinization. (× 5)

FIGURE 109. *Case 20:* Ovary at autopsy 23 months after a hydatidiform mole, showing a theca-lutein cyst and ectopic decidual plaques (see FIGURE 98). (× 39)

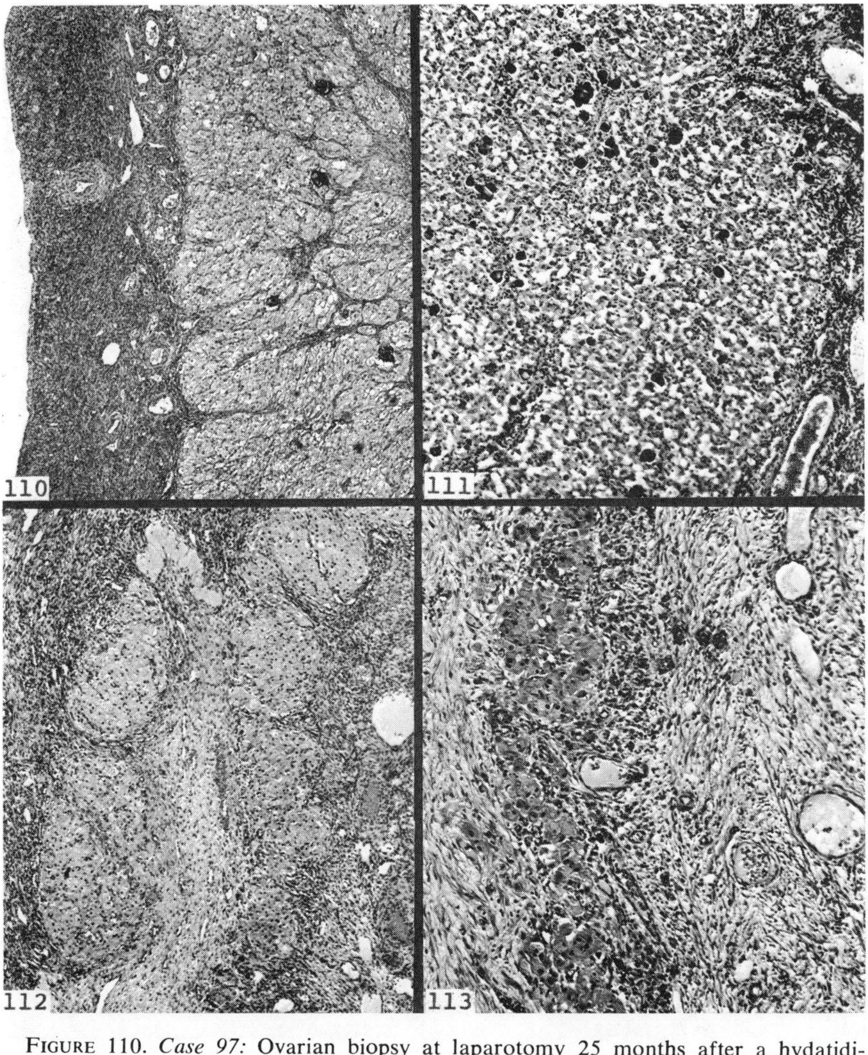

FIGURE 110. *Case 97:* Ovarian biopsy at laparotomy 25 months after a hydatidiform mole, showing diffuse stromal luteinization with calcospherites. (× 36)

FIGURE 111. *Case 3:* Ovary at autopsy 10 months postpartum, showing a luteinized structure with scattered calcospherites. (× 56)

FIGURE 112. *Case 38:* Ovary at laparotomy 10 weeks after an abortion, showing nodular configuration of luteinized theca around an atretic follicle. (× 42)

FIGURE 113. *Case 38:* Another field from same slide as in FIGURE 112, showing stromal luteinization. (× 80)

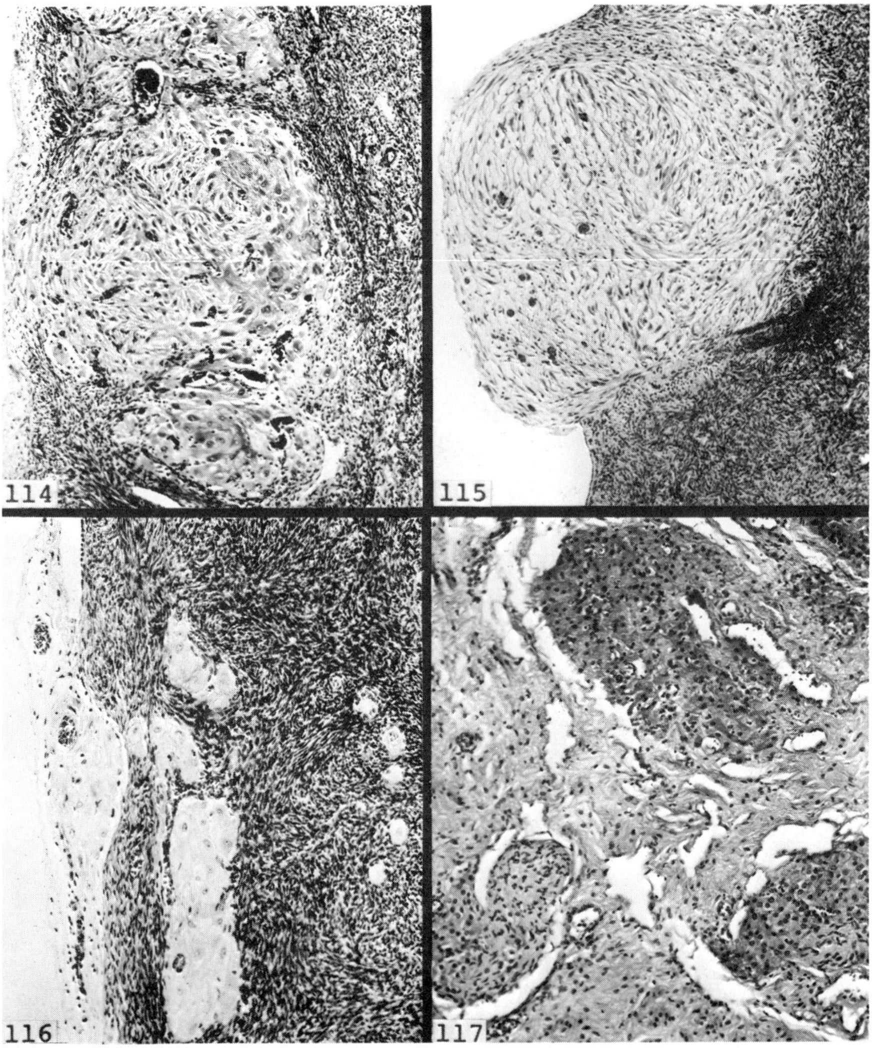

FIGURE 114. *Case 3:* Ovary at autopsy 10 months postpartum, showing a plaque of ectopic decidua in the subcoelomic mesenchyme. The HCG titer was >4,000,000 units. (× 64)

FIGURE 115. *Case 15:* Ovary at autopsy 12 months after term delivery, showing a plaque of ectopic decidua at the cortical surface (see FIGURE 105) (× 72)

FIGURE 116. *Case 1:* Ovary at autopsy 1 year after delivery, showing ectopic decidua on and just below the surface as well as in a delicate periovarian adhesion (see FIGURE 104). (× 102)

FIGURE 117. *Case 27:* Ovary at autopsy 26 months after a hydatidiform mole, showing nests of hyperplastic hilar cells. (× 85)

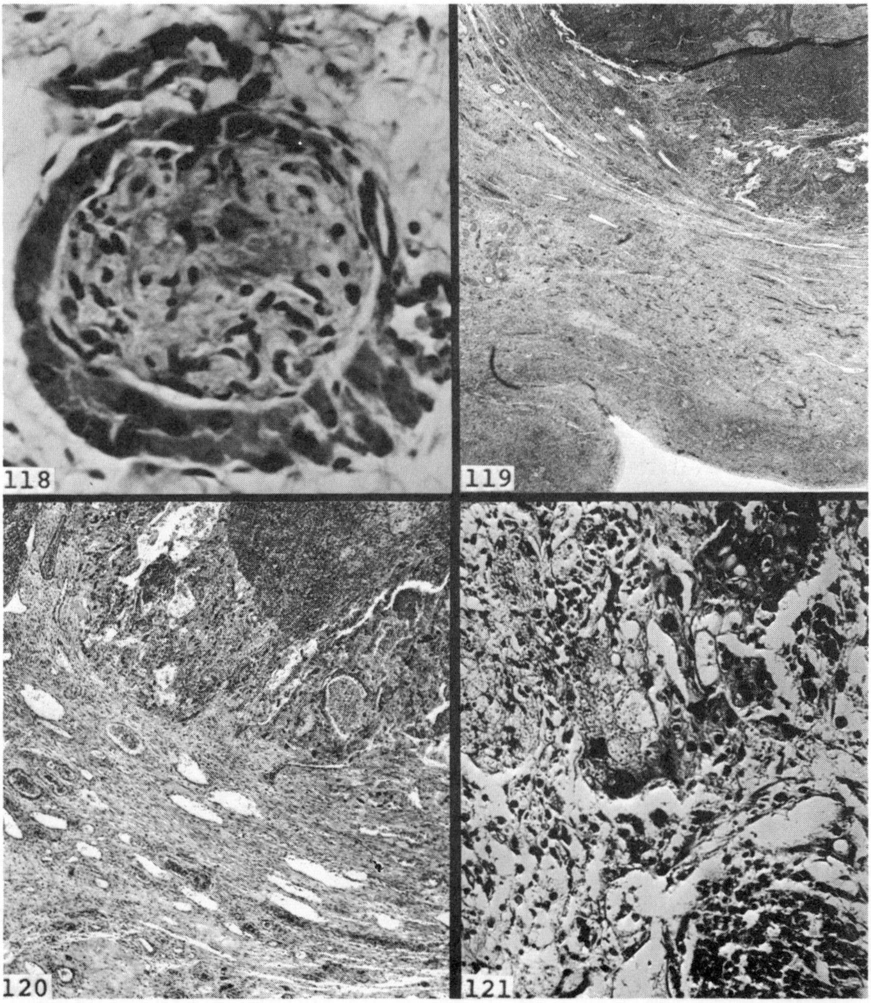

FIGURE 118. *Case 15:* Ovary at autopsy 12 months after term delivery, showing a collar of hilar cells around as small nerve bundle. (see FIGURES 105 & 115). (× 357)

FIGURE 119. *Case 34:* Ovary at autopsy 40 months after a hydatidiform mole, showing metastatic choriocarcinoma with hemorrhage. (× 15)

FIGURE 120. *Case 34:* Detail of FIGURE 119, showing the rim of viable choriocarcinoma abutting ovarian medulla. (× 31)

FIGURE 121. *Case 51:* Tumor of the right ovary, showing vacuolated plasmodia of syncytiotrophoblast in a matrix of poorly differentiated embryonal cells. (× 136)

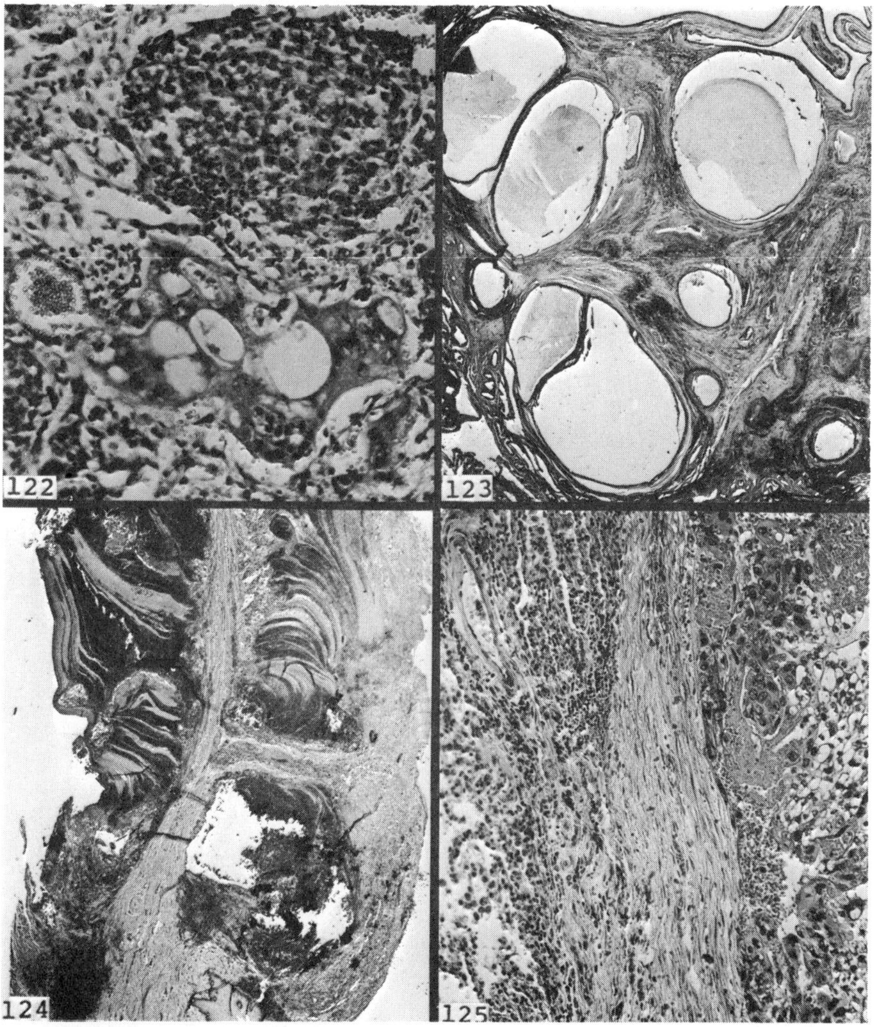

FIGURE 122. *Case 51:* A nearby field in the same slide as FIGURE 121, showing a syncytiotrophoblastic plasmodium next to a nest of immature, reticular cells resembling cytotrophoblast. (× 119)

FIGURE 123. *Case 51:* Left ovary showing many cystically dilated follicles with no evidence of luteinization. (× 4)

FIGURE 124. *Case 52:* Vaginal metastasis at autopsy 6 weeks after laparotomy, showing metastatic choriocarcinoma with ulceration, necrosis, and hemorrhage. (× 8.5)

FIGURE 125. *Case 52:* Left adnexal mass, showing a tumor composed of both disgerminomatous and choriocarcinomatous elements. (× 85)

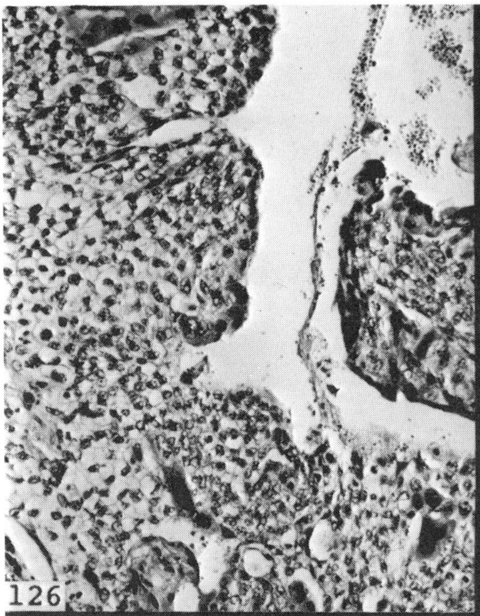

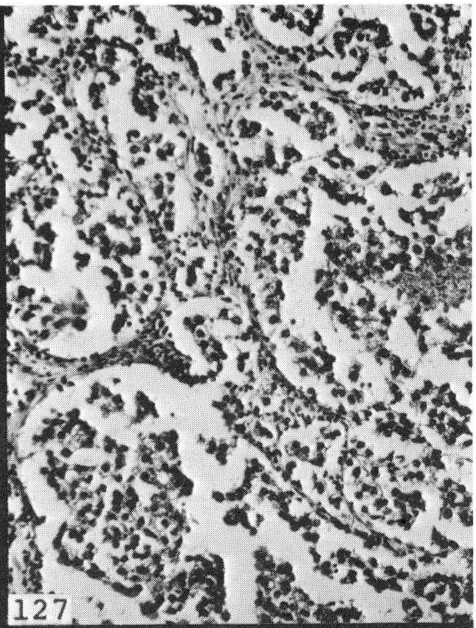

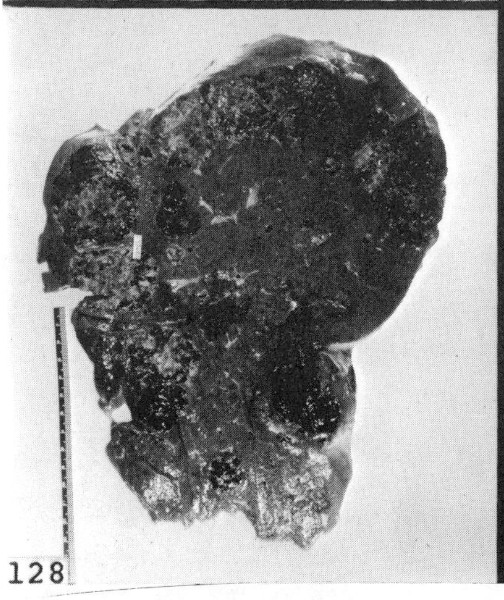

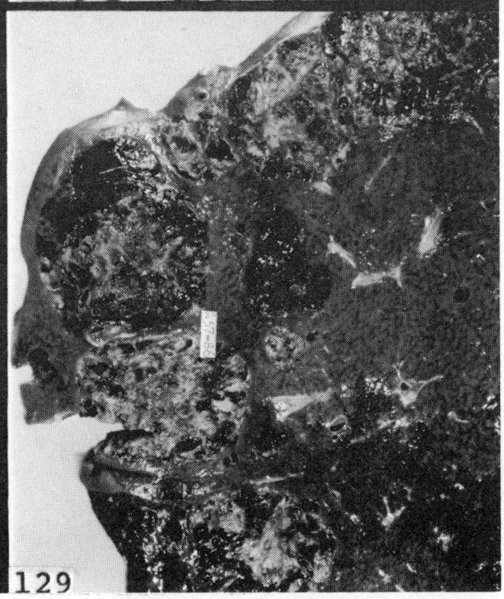

FIGURE 126. *Case 52:* Detail of FIGURE 125, showing choriocarcinoma, (× 122)

FIGURE 127. *Case 52:* Detail of FIGURE 125, showing disgerminoma. (× 99)

FIGURE 128. *Case 52:* Liver at autopsy 6 weeks after laparotomy, showing multiple nodules of metastatic choriocarcinoma with hemorrhage and necrosis.

FIGURE 129. *Case 52:* Close-up view of liver, showing the hemorrhagic nodules of metastatic choriocarcinoma just beneath Glisson's capsule at the inferior margin of the liver.

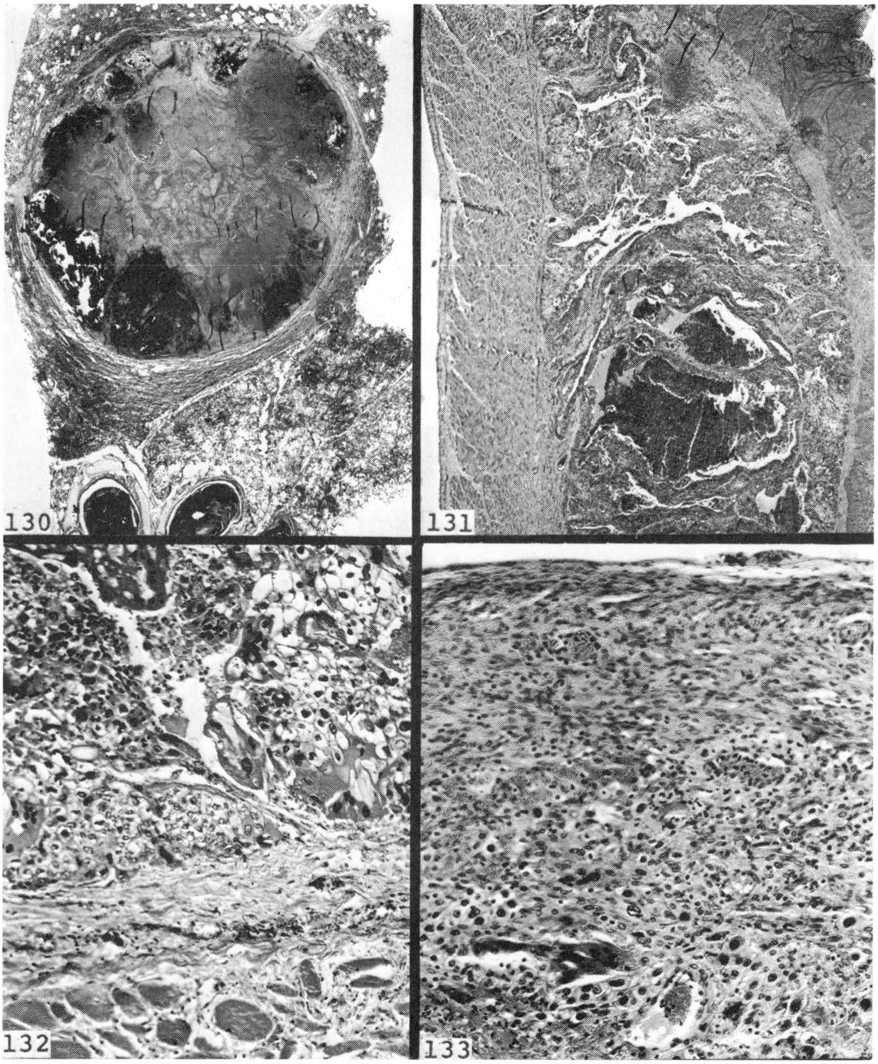

FIGURE 130. *Case 52:* Lung at autopsy 6 weeks after laparotomy, showing a hemorrhagic nodule of metastatic choriocarcinoma. Thrombi are present in branches of the pulmonary artery. (× 3.4)

FIGURE 131. *Case 52:* Choriocarcinoma metastatic to the diaphragm, covered by a layer of fibrin. (× 9)

FIGURE 132. *Case 52:* Detail of FIGURE 131, showing vacuolated syncytiotrophoblast in the diaphragmatic metastasis. (× 94)

FIGURE 133. *Case 52:* Left ovary with a complex neoplasm containing choriocarcinomatous elements. (× 106)

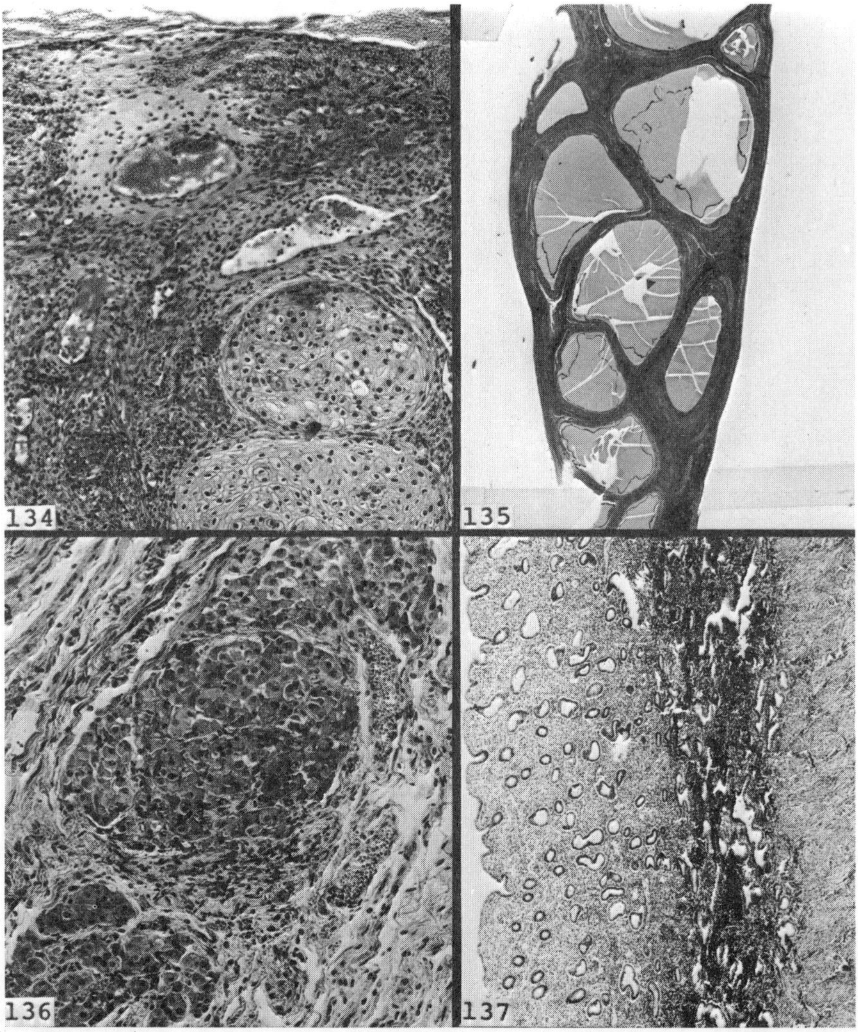

FIGURE 134. *Case 52:* Complex neoplasm in the left ovary, showing teratoid elements. (× 81)

FIGURE 135. *Case 52:* Right ovary 13 months after removal of an ovarian teratocarcinoma, showing multiple cystically expanded follicles filled with coagulated liquor folliculi. There is no increase of granulosa cells or theca interna. (× 4)

FIGURE 136. *Case 52:* Hilus of right ovary, showing hyperplasia of hilar cells. (× 128)

FIGURE 137. *Case 52:* Uterus at autopsy 13 months after removal of an ovarian teratocarcinoma with choriocarcinomatous elements. The endometrial glands are slightly coiled, but there is no secretion or mitotic activity; the stroma is inactive, and the arterioles are undeveloped. The remaining ovary showed follicular cysts and hilus cell hyperplasia. (× 24)

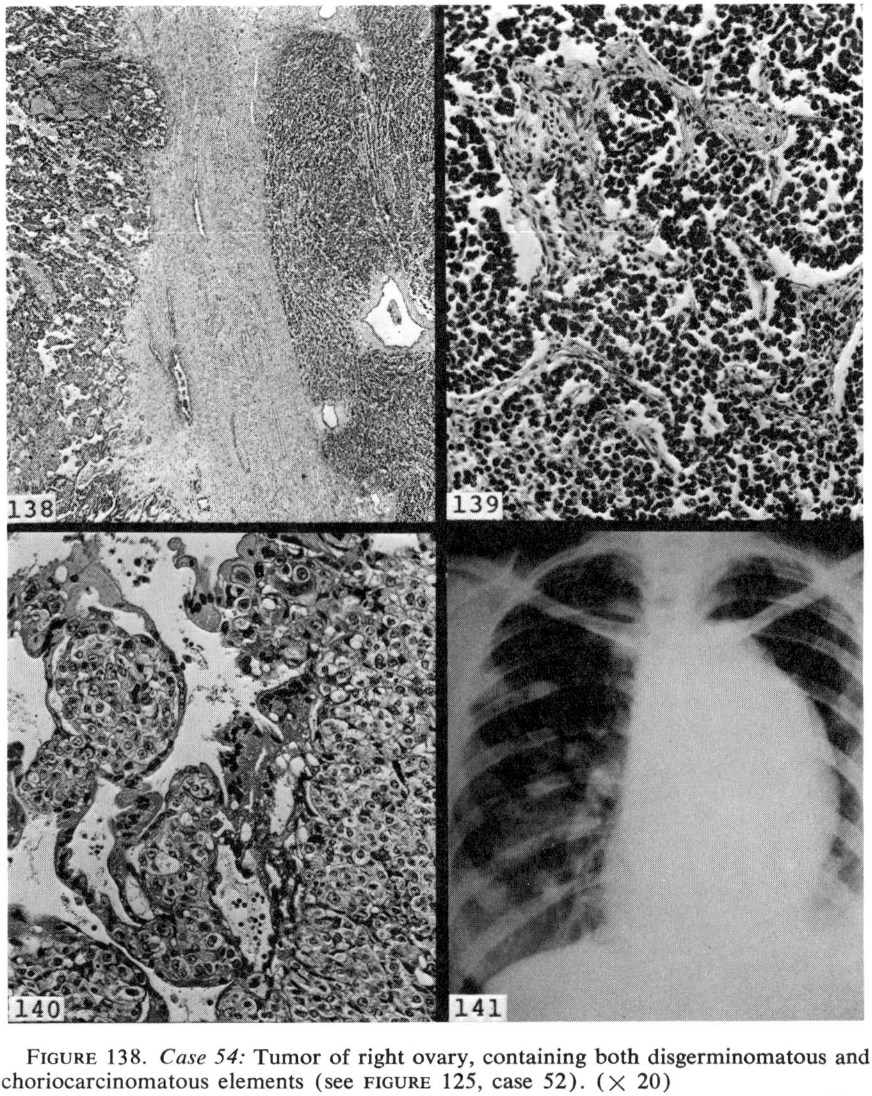

FIGURE 138. *Case 54:* Tumor of right ovary, containing both disgerminomatous and choriocarcinomatous elements (see FIGURE 125, case 52). (× 20)

FIGURE 139. *Case 54:* Detail of FIGURE 138, showing disgerminoma. (× 115)

FIGURE 140. *Case 54:* Detail of FIGURE 138, showing choriocarcinoma. (× 115)

FIGURE 141. *Case 47:* Chest x-ray on admission 11 months after a spontaneous abortion, showing multiple nodular densities in the right lung and a large mass overlying the left cardiac border. The patient died 1 week later, but permission for autopsy could not be obtained.

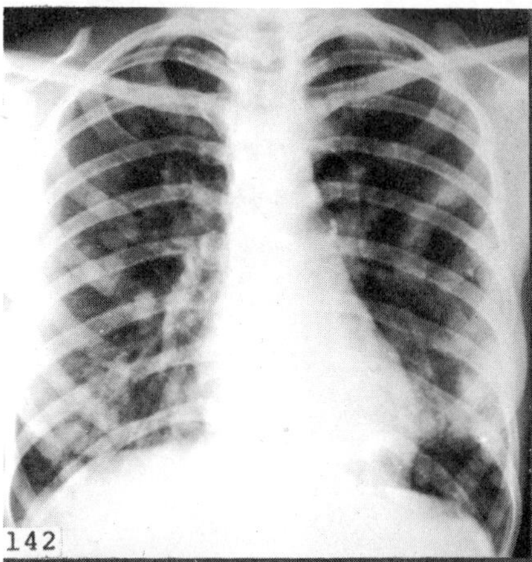

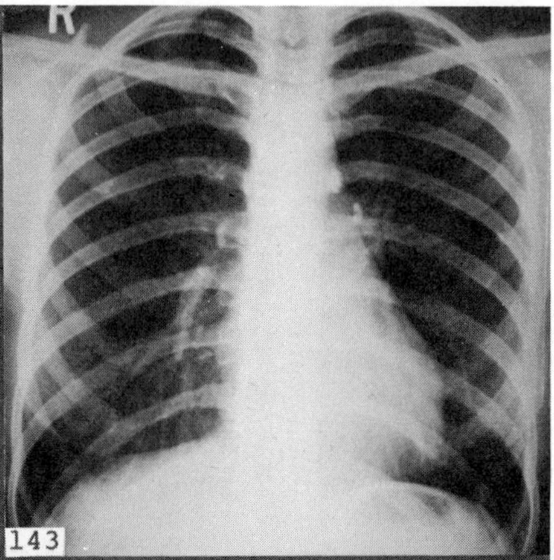

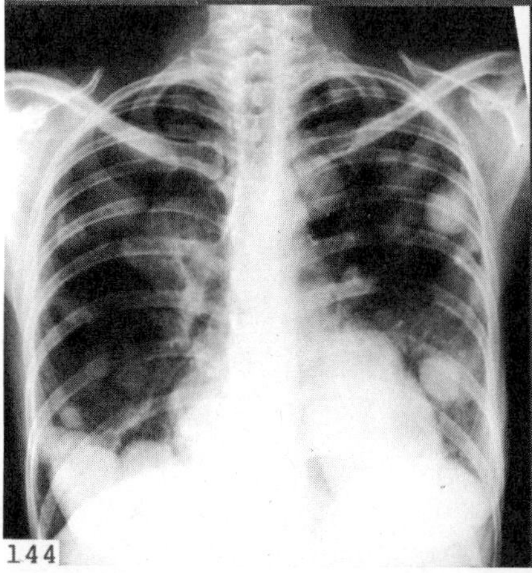

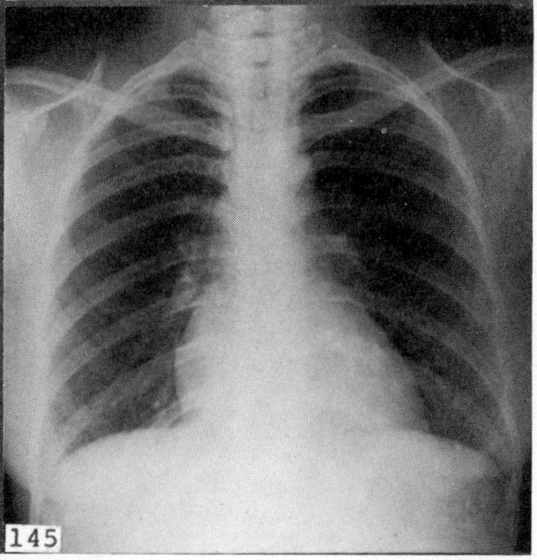

FIGURE 142. *Case 77:* Chest x-ray on admission 5.5 months after a hydatidiform mole, showing multiple nodular densities in both lung fields (see FIGURES 15–17).

FIGURE 143. *Case 77:* Chest x-ray 16 months after admission, showing clearing of all lesions after four courses of methotrexate.

FIGURE 144. *Case 89:* Chest roentgenogram on admission 6 months after spontaneous abortion showing nodular densities in both lung fields.

FIGURE 145. *Case 89:* Chest x-ray 14 months after hysterectomy for invasive choriocarcinoma, showing clear lung fields. Patient had received six courses of methotrexate, three of vincaleukoblastine, and three of actinomycin-D.

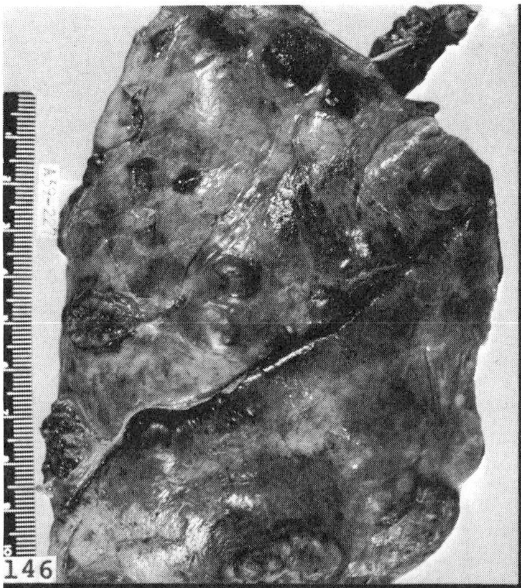

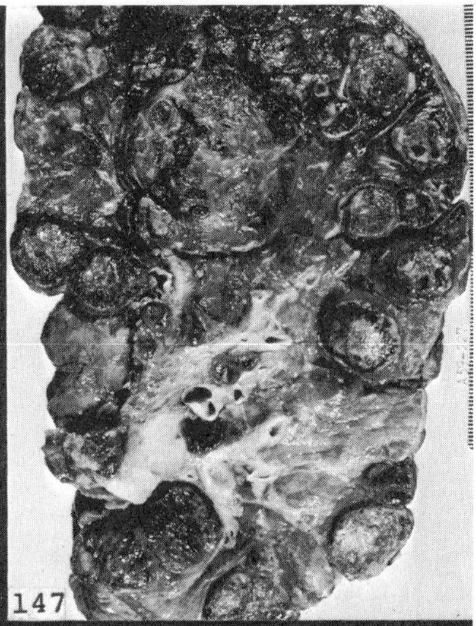

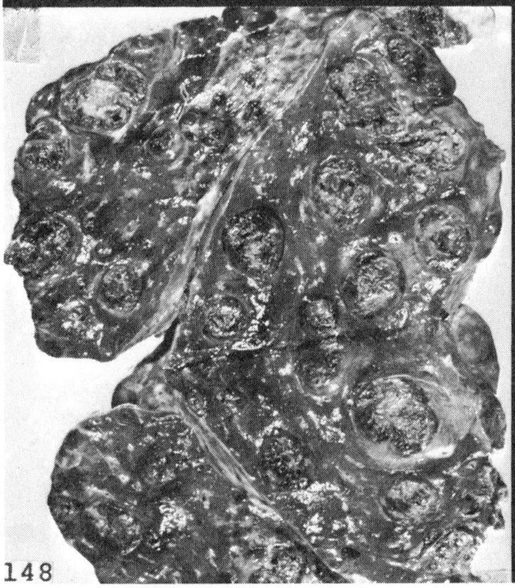

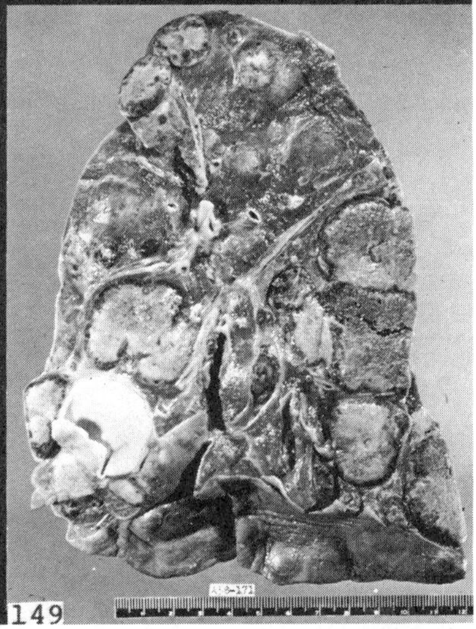

FIGURE 146. *Case 40:* Pleural surface of the left lung at autopsy 11 months after a spontaneous abortion. The lung parenchyma is extensively replaced by nodules of metastatic choriocarcinoma up to 4 cm in diameter. Patient received seven courses of methotrexate, four of vincaleukoblastine, and two of cyclophosphamide.

FIGURE 147. *Case 40:* Cut surface of the left lung (see FIGURE 146), showing appearance of metastatic nodules with necrotic centers replacing over 75% of pulmonary parenchyma.

FIGURE 148. *Case 9:* Left lung at autopsy 8 months after term delivery, showing over 30 metastatic nodules, 1–3 cm in diameter (see FIGURES 18, 19, & 92).

FIGURE 149. *Case 1:* Cut surface of the lung at autopsy 1 year after term delivery, showing many metastatic deposits of choriocarcinoma. The largest nodules were 3 cm in diameter and showed extensive central necrosis.

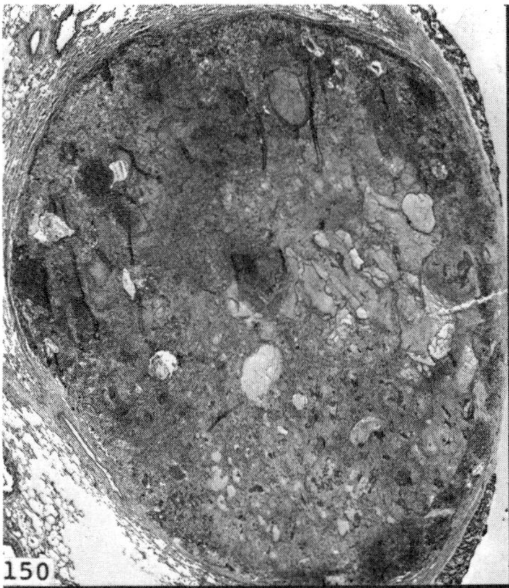

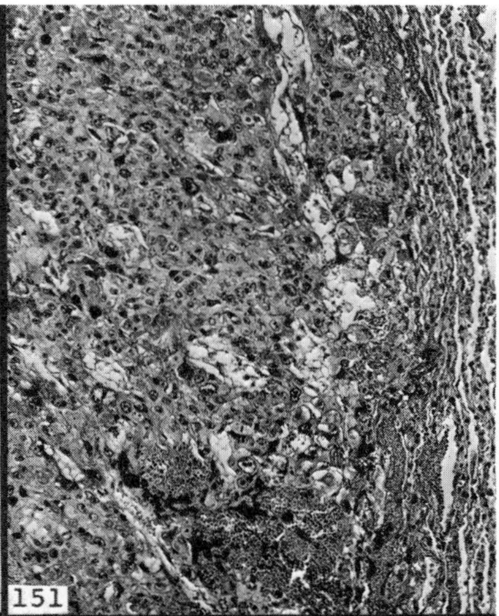

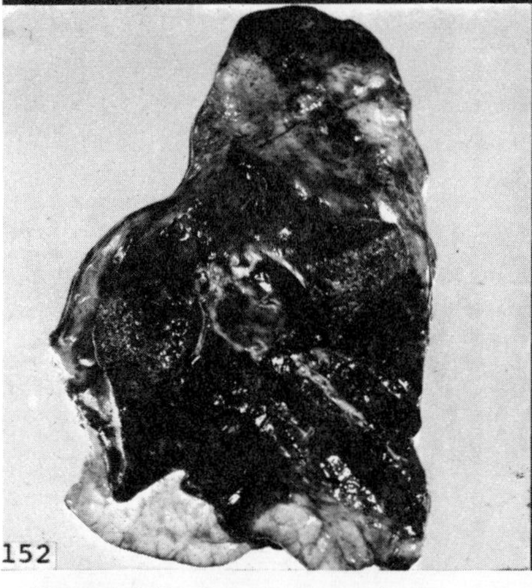

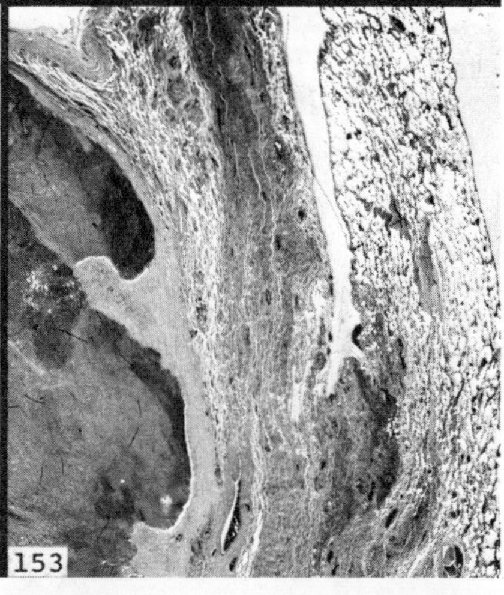

FIGURE 150. *Case 1:* Lung 1 year post partum, showing a subpleural deposit of choriocarcinoma which is largely necrotic. Fibrinous pleuritis is also present. (× 8)

FIGURE 151. *Case 1:* Lung 1 year after term delivery, showing viable metastatic choriocarcinoma after five courses of methotrexate and additional chemotherapy. (X 81)

FIGURE 152. *Case 20:* Lower lobe of the right lung removed at thoracotomy 1 year after a hydatidiform mole. This solitary 3-cm metastatic nodule did not regress after five courses of methotrexate and two of vincaleukoblastine. The patient died 11 months after lobectomy, with multiple intrapulmonic metastases, a solitary cerebral metastasis, and other secondary deposits elsewhere.

FIGURE 153. *Case 20:* The nodule shown in FIGURE 152 is surrounded by a zone of compressed lung tissue, and a hyaline wall has formed. Much of the nodule is necrotic; no viable trophoblast is present in the area shown. (× 4) Lobectomy was performed when additional methotrexate and vincaleukoblastine failed to reduce the size of the nodule or the level of the HCG titer after a period of initial improvement.

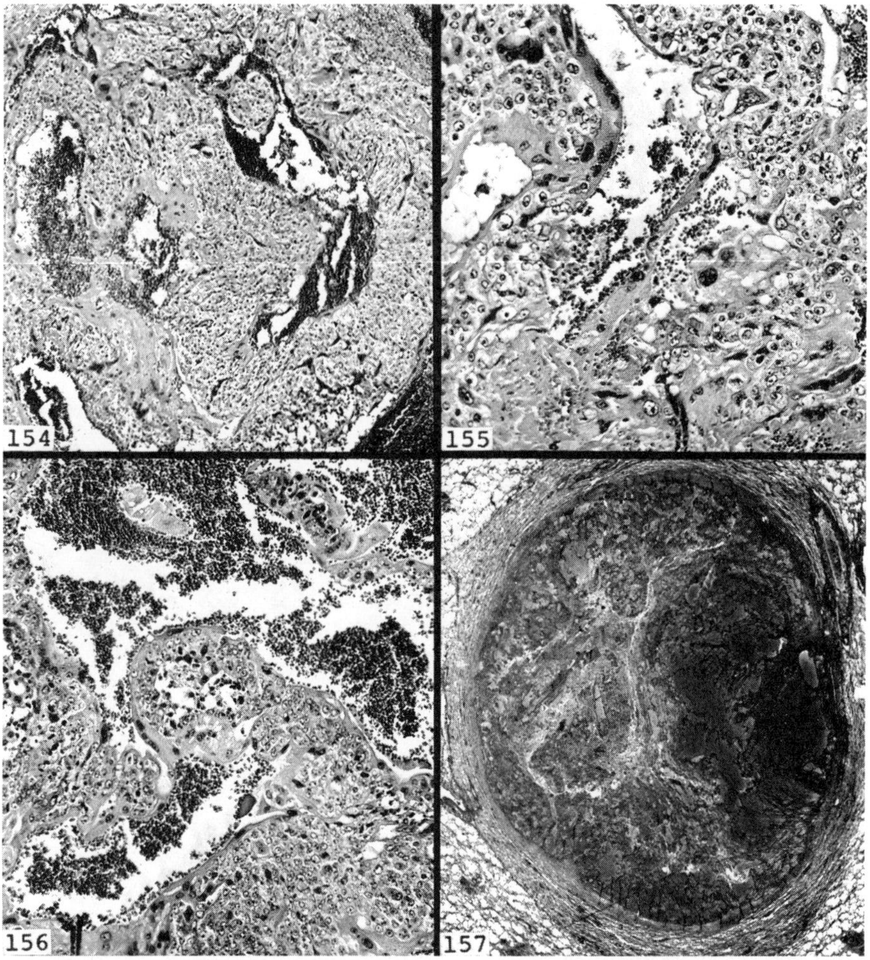

FIGURE 154. *Case 20:* Field in center of the pulmonary nodule shown in FIGURE 153, showing viable trophoblast surrounded by hemorrhage and necrosis. Sinusoidal lacunae within the mass of trophoblast are lined by flattened syncytiotrophoblast and represent the course of intrinsic circulation within the secondary deposit. (× 47)

FIGURE 155. *Case 20:* Detail of FIGURE 154, showing sinusoids lined by syncytiotrophoblast one cell layer thick, and fresh hemorrhage at the point where attenuated syncytiotrophoblast has disappeared. (× 86)

FIGURE 156. *Case 20:* Detail of FIGURE 154, showing sinusoids lined by syncytiotrophoblast of variable thickness, and destruction of tumor by hemorrhage. (× 108)

FIGURE 157. *Case 6:* Lung 6 months postpartum, showing a large hemorrhagic metastasis of uterine choriocarcinoma. Early bronchopneumonia is present in the lung parenchyma around the tumor, and *Staphylococcus aureus* was recovered from the blood. (× 5)

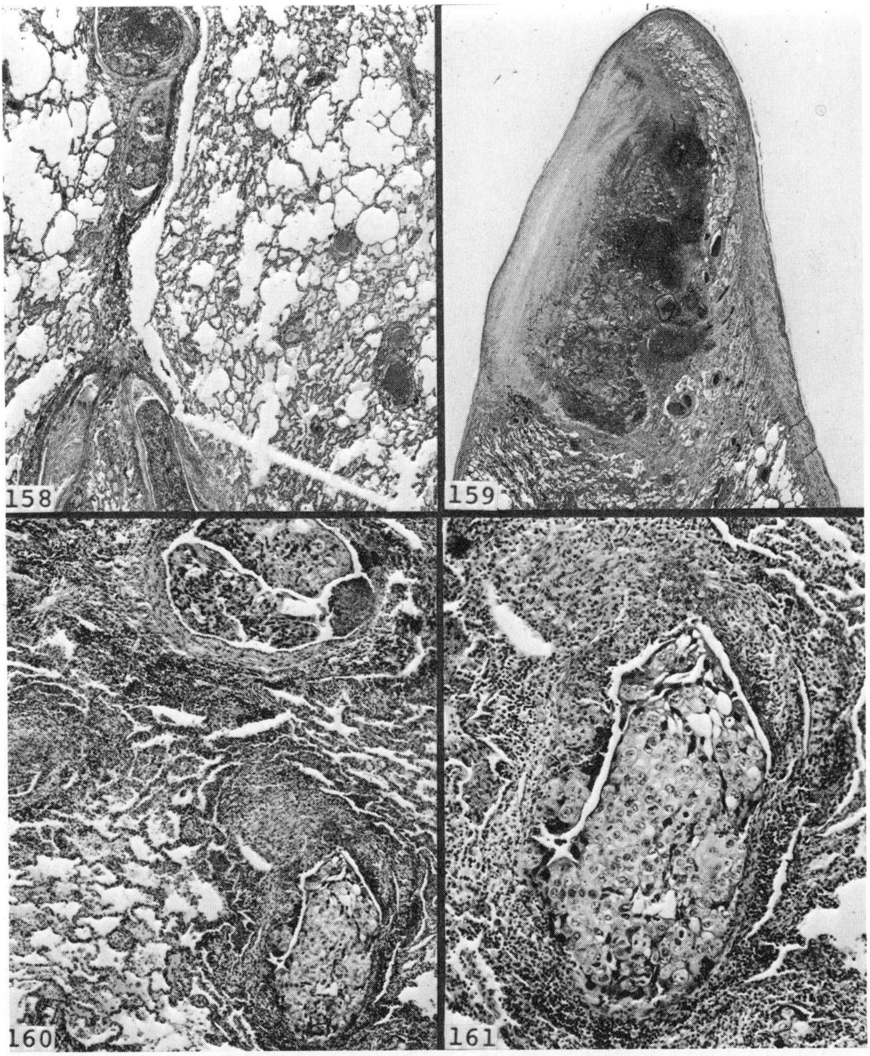

FIGURE 158. *Case 4:* Lung in an untreated patient 8 months after term delivery, showing emboli of neoplastic trophoblast in branches of the pulmonary artery tree (see FIGURE 85.) (× 17)

FIGURE 159. *Case 4:* Lung in an untreated patient, showing a marginal pulmonary infarct and a thrombus in the supplying arterial ramus. Although extensive metastases of choriocarcinoma were present in other portions of the lung, not all roentgenographically demonstrated lesions are metastases. (× 7)

FIGURE 160. *Case 80:* Lung at lobectomy 9 years after a hydatidiform mole, showing embolic neoplastic trophoblast within medium-sized vessels surrounded by an inflammatory reaction sufficiently large to produce a radiologically visible shadow and a positive HCG titer. (× 43)

FIGURE 161. *Case 80:* Detail of FIGURE 160. (× 85)

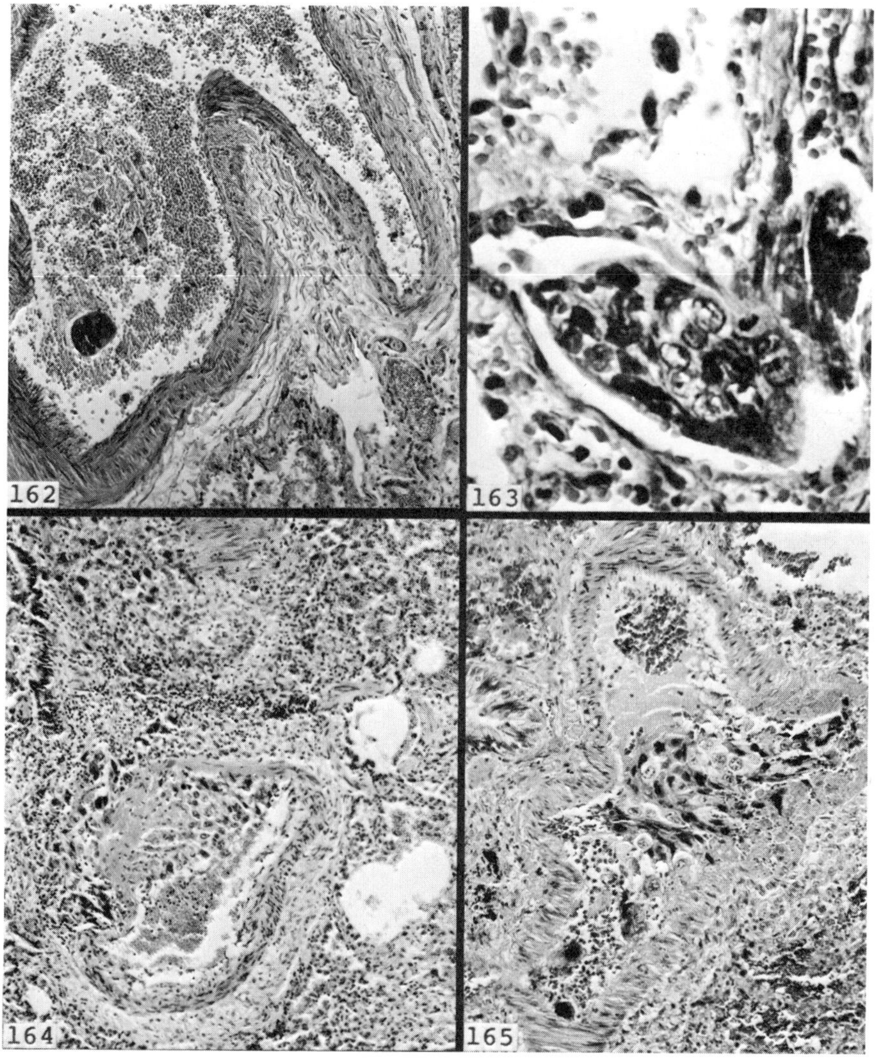

FIGURE 162. *Case 21:* Lung 5 months after a hydatidiform mole in an essentially untreated patient, showing small emboli of trophoblast in large branches of the pulmonary artery. (× 92)

FIGURE 163. *Case 3:* Lung 10 months postpartum, showing embolic syncytiotrophoblast in a small intrapulmonic vessel. (× 323)

FIGURE 164. *Case 38:* Lung 10 months after an abortion, showing embolic choriocarcinoma migrating into lung parenchyma through a necrotic segment of the wall of a small artery. (× 72)

FIGURE 165. *Case 38:* Pulmonary blood vessel showing segmental necrosis; perivascular inflammation is minimal. (× 106)

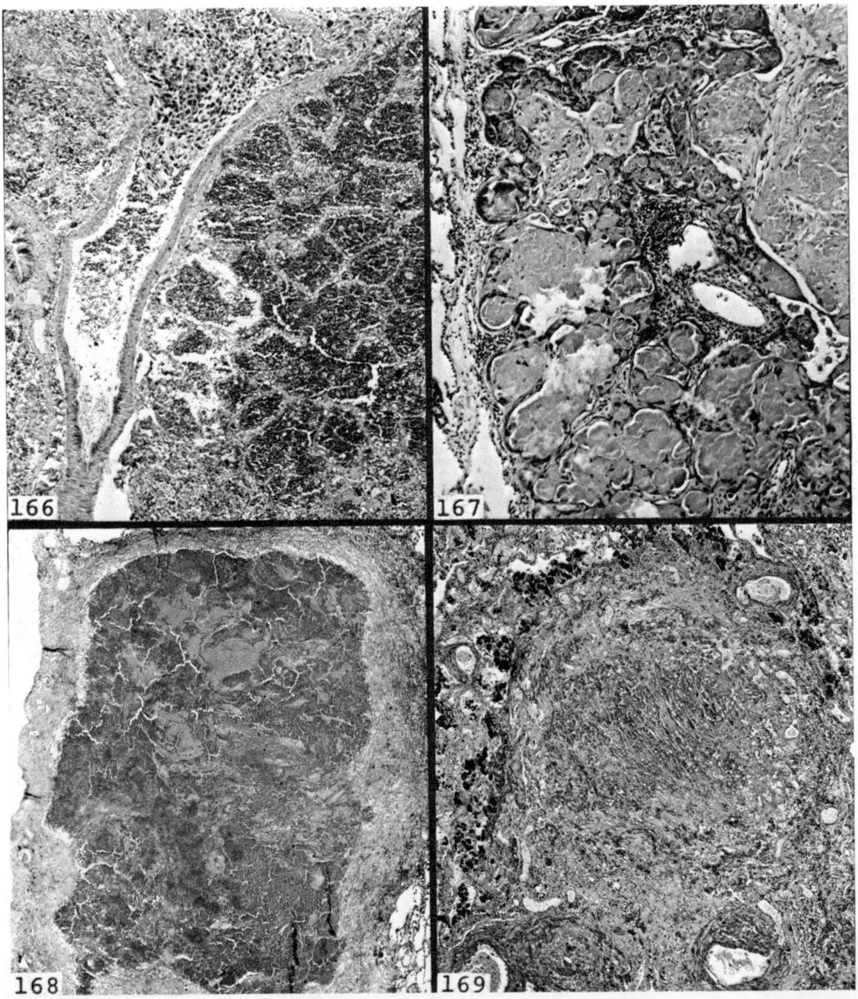

FIGURE 166. *Case 38:* Lung 10 months after an abortion in an untreated patient dying with obstructive pulmonary hypertension, showing embolic choriocarcinoma and thrombus occluding a medium-sized artery, with infarction of the subtended pulmonary parenchyma. (× 38)

FIGURE 167. *Case 22:* Lung biopsy 10 months after a hydatidiform mole, showing a nodule of metastatic choriocarcinoma. The cytotrophoblast has undergone spontaneous necrosis, leaving syncytiotrophoblast in a crescentic configuration around the eosinophilic debris. (× 60)

FIGURE 168. *Case 16:* Lung 23 months postpartum, showing a secondary deposit that is entirely necrotic, without viable trophoblast, after five courses of methotrexate and five of actinomycin-D The patient died of hemorrhage from a cerebral metastasis (see FIGURE 91). (× 14)

FIGURE 169. *Case 37:* Lung 8 months after an abortion. Following one course of methotrexate, the pulmonary nodules were almost completely necrotic, but surrounded by colonies of bacteria. (× 30)

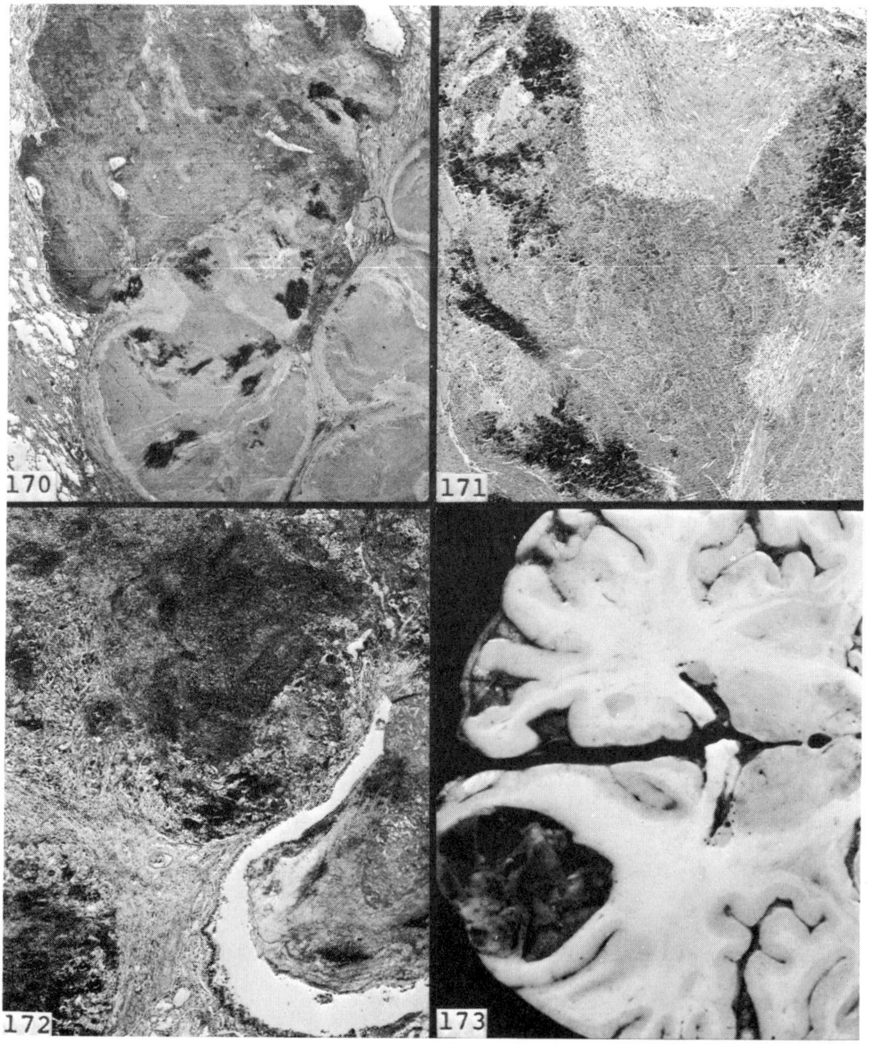

FIGURE 170. *Case 17:* Lung 14 months postpartum, showing extensive necrosis and calcification of secondary choriocarcinoma. Only minute foci of viable trophoblast remain in the lungs. The patient died of intraperitoneal hemorrhage from a ruptured liver metastasis. (× 10)

FIGURE 171. *Case 17:* Detail of FIGURE 170, showing calcification. (× 31)

FIGURE 172. *Case 5:* Lung 7 months postpartum, showing metastatic choriocarcinoma with hemorrhage rupturing into a bronchus (see FIGURE 59). (× 17)

FIGURE 173. *Case 23:* Coronal section of the brain 15 months after a hydatidiform mole, showing a solitary 4-cm metastatic nodule of hemorrhage choriocarcinoma in the right parietal lobe.

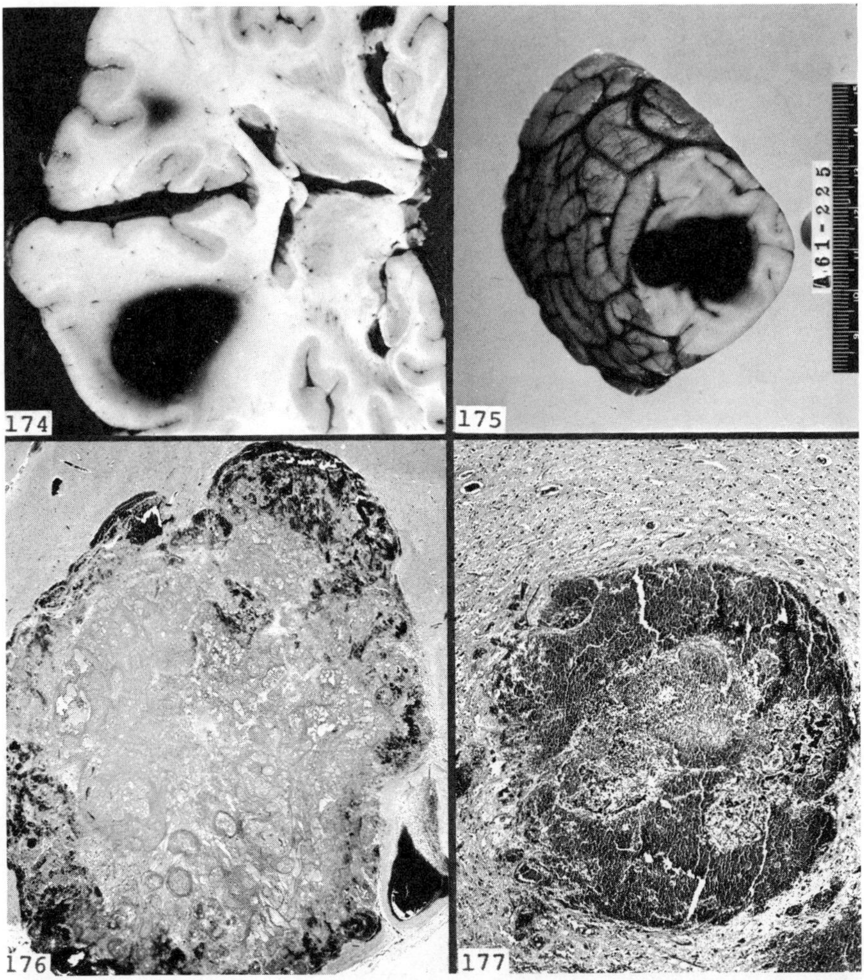

FIGURE 174. *Case 29:* Coronal section of the brain 4 years after a hydatidiform mole, showing multiple hemorrhagic areas in the white matter associated with metastatic deposits of choriocarcinoma.

FIG. 175. *Case 34:* Brain 40 months after a hydatidiform mole, showing a hemorrhagic nodule of metastatic choriocarcinoma in the occipital lobe, with hemorrhage into the lateral ventricle.

FIGURE 176. *Case 27:* Cerebral cortex 26 months after a hydatidiform mole, showing a module of metastatic choriocarcinoma in the center of a gyrus. The center of the nodule is necrotic; only a thin rim of viable trophoblast persists at the periphery. The overlying pia-arachnoid is adherent. An adjacent blood vessel is distended by a partially organized thrombus. (× 5)

FIGURE 177. *Case 42:* Small intracerebral metastasis of choriocarcinoma 24 months after an abortion. Fresh hemorrhage is more abundant than the volume of neoplastic trophoblast. (× 25)

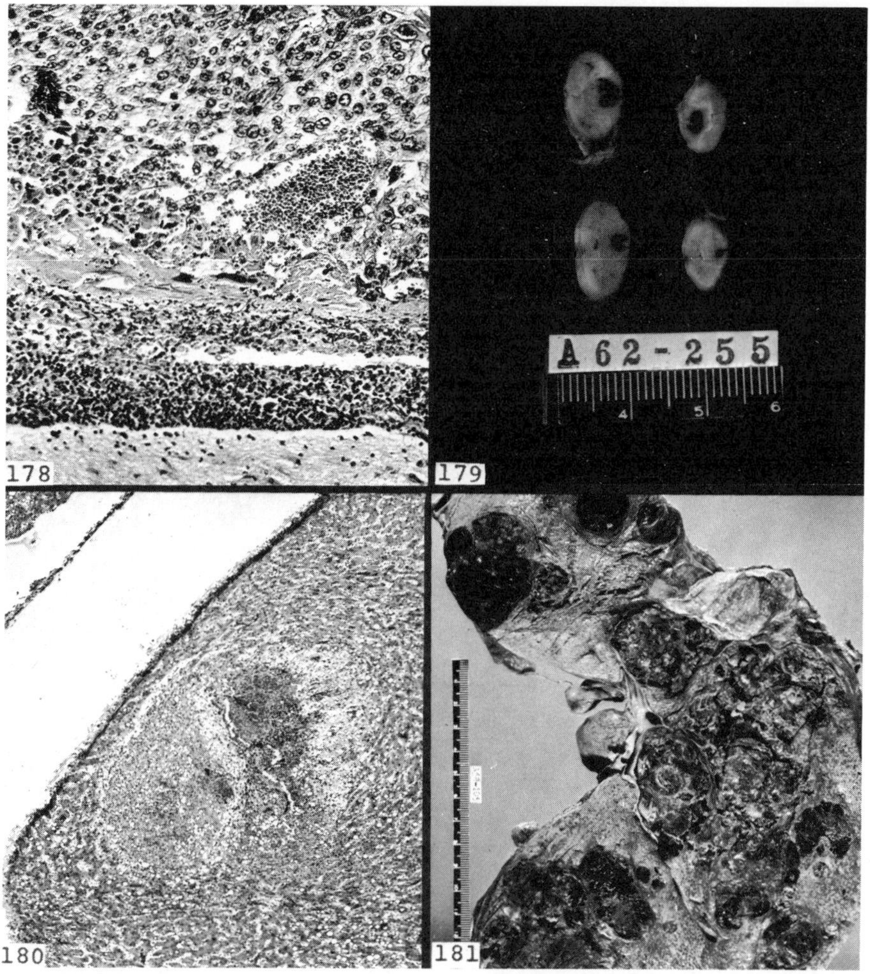

FIGURE 178. *Case 2:* Cerebral cortex, showing metastatic choriocarcinoma separated from brain tissue by a thin layer of hemorrhage. (× 108)

FIGURE 179. *Case 41:* Sections of spinal cord 14 months after a spontaneous abortion, showing foci of hemorrhagic necrosis associated with metastatic choriocarcinoma.

FIGURE 180. *Case 42:* Liver 24 months after an abortion, showing a small hemorrhagic deposit of choriocarcinoma abutting a major intrahepatic duct. Only minimal fatty vacuolation is seen in liver cells despite three courses of methotrexate, the last two in high dosage, five courses of vincaleukoblastine, three of actinomycin-D, and five of "triple therapy." (× 26)

FIGURE 181. *Case 21:* Cut surface of the liver 5 months after a hydatidiform mole, showing multiple large confluent metastases of choriocarcinoma, many of which are hemorrhagic. Death was due to rupture of one of them, with massive hemoperitoneum.

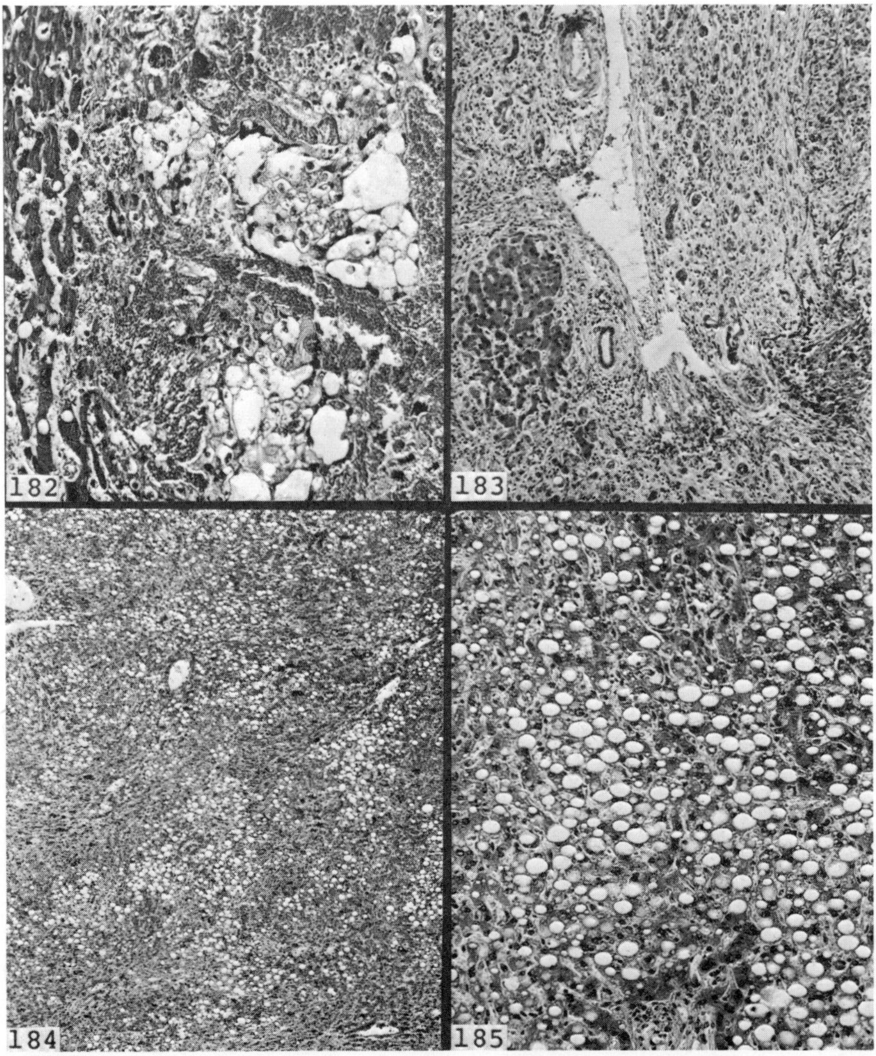

FIGURE 182. *Case 21:* Liver 5 months after a hydatidiform mole, showing metastatic choriocarcinoma with hemorrhage and vacuolation of syncytiotrophoblast (see FIGURE 181). (× 113)

FIGURE 183. *Case 29:* Liver 4 years after a hydatidiform mole, showing severe postnecrotic scarring and a sheet of metastatic choriocarcinoma. (× 68)

FIGURE 184. *Case 34:* Liver 40 months after a hydatidiform mole and three courses of methotrexate, three of actinomycin-D, and four of actinomycin-D with chlorambucil, showing diffuse fatty metamorphosis. (× 23)

FIGURE 185. *Case 5:* Liver 7 months after term delivery and four courses of methotrexate during the 2 months before death, showing diffuse fatty metamorphosis. (× 97)

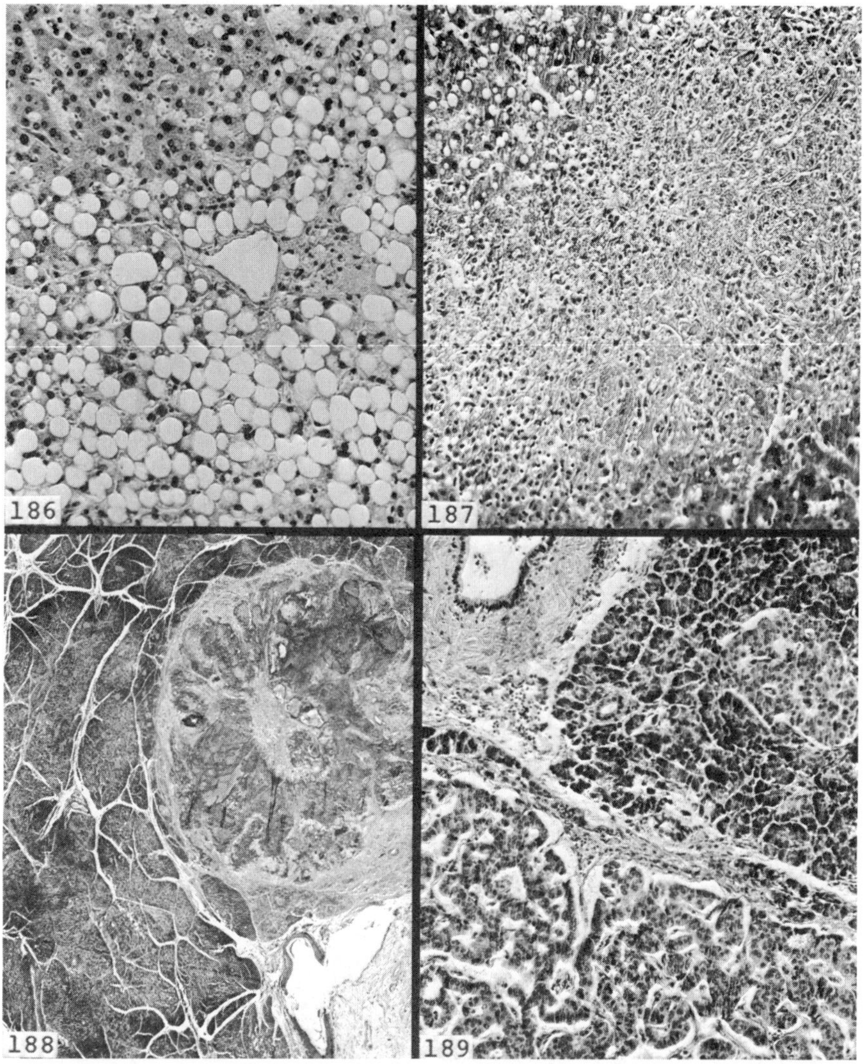

FIGURE 186. *Case 44:* Liver 5 months after choriocarcinoma was diagnosed by biopsy of a labium minus, showing severe fatty metamorphosis and small foci of paracentral necrosis. Patient received four courses of "triple therapy" and one of actinomycin-D. (× 170)

FIGURE 187. *Case 21:* Liver 5 months after a hydatidiform mole and one course of methotrexate, showing moderate fatty metamorphosis and zonal necrosis (see FIGURES 181 & 182). (× 102)

FIGURE 188. *Case 27:* Pancreas 26 months after a hydatidiform mole, showing a metastatic nodule of choriocarcinoma. A zone of central necrosis is surrounded by a circumferential zone of hemorrhage, and the only viable trophoblast forms a thin rim abutting the pancreatic parenchyma. (× 5)

FIGURE 189. *Case 28:* Pancreas at autopsy 10 months after a hydatidiform mole, showing a well-circumscribed islet-cell adenoma. There was no clinical or laboratory evidence of hypoglycemia. (× 102)

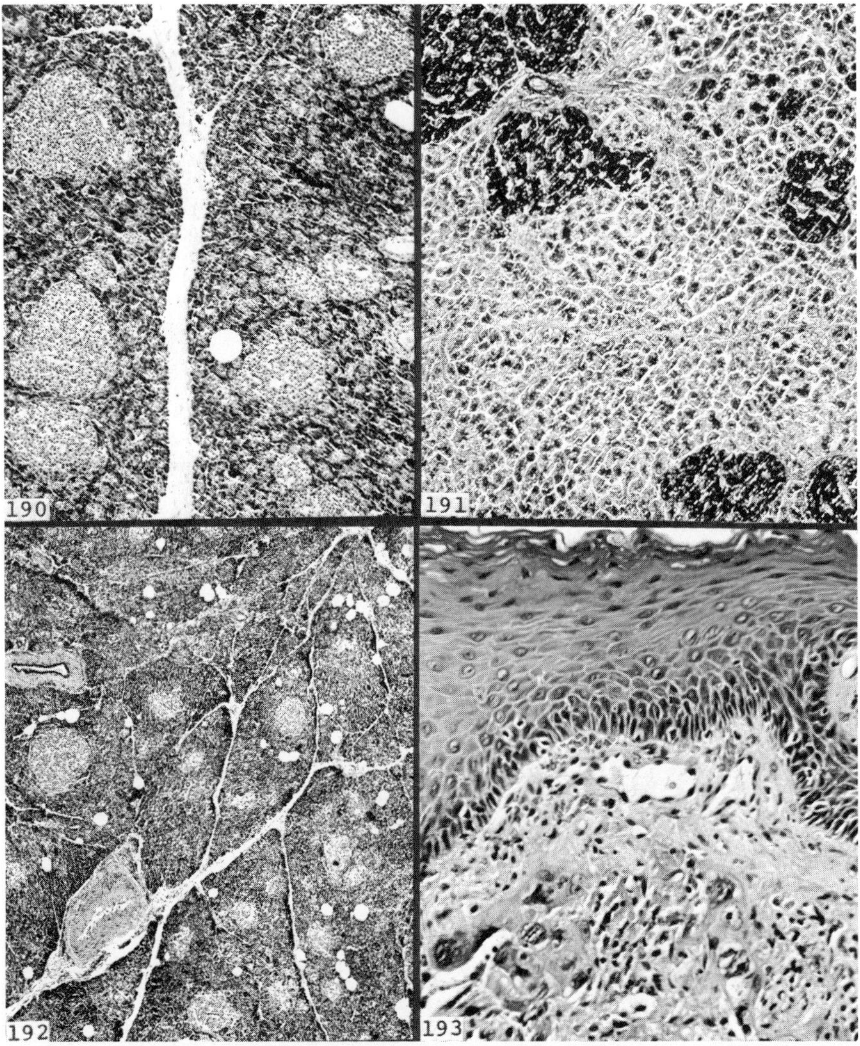

FIGURE 190. *Case 28:* Pancreas 10 months after a hydatidiform mole, showing moderate increase in number and size of islets of Langerhans (see FIGURE 189). (× 49)

FIGURE 191. *Case 33:* Pancreas 35 months after a hydatidiform mole, showing moderate increase in number and size of islets of Langerhans. Stain: Gaulin-Krasnopolsky. (× 71)

FIGURE 192. *Case 35:* Pancreas 23 months after a hydatidiform mole, showing moderate increase in number and size of islets of Langerhans. (× 23)

FIGURE 193. *Case 34:* Biopsy of gingiva 3 years after a hydatidiform mole, showing permeation of submucosa by trophoblast. The lesion resembles a regressing vaginal nodule. (× 150)

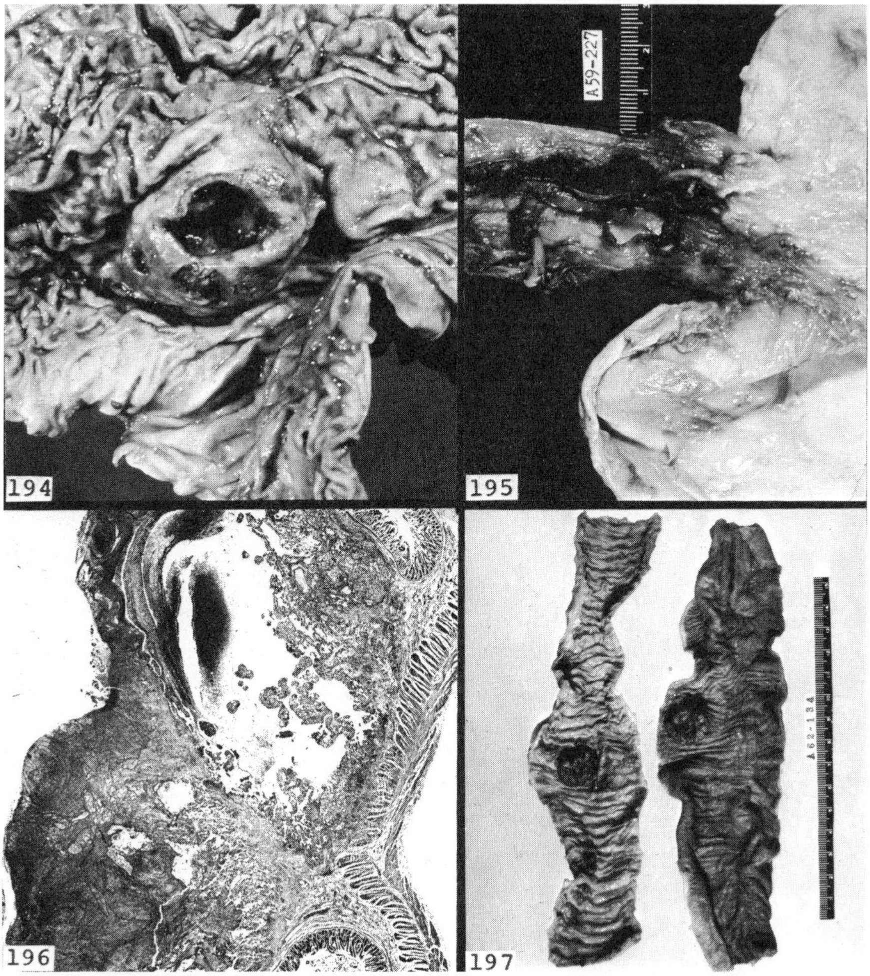

FIGURE 194. *Case 1:* Stomach at autopsy 1 year after term delivery, showing an elevated intramural nodule of metastatic choriocarcinoma with an ulcerated center.

FIGURE 195. *Case 40:* Terminal esophagus at autopsy 11 months after a spontaneous abortion, showing linear rupture into the mediastinum. The patient developed severe vomiting after seven courses of methotrexate, four of vincaleukoblastine, and two of cyclophosphamide.

FIGURE 196. *Case 3:* Small intestine 10 months postpartum, showing metastatic choriocarcinoma in the submucosa, with perforation of mucosa producing massive gastrintestinal bleeding. ($\times$ 6)

FIGURE 197. *Case 30:* Segments of small intestine at autopsy 46 months after a hydatidiform mole, showing two sharply marginated, ulcerated deposits of choriocarcinoma. Tertiary deposits were found in mesenteric lymph nodes draining these segments of bowel.

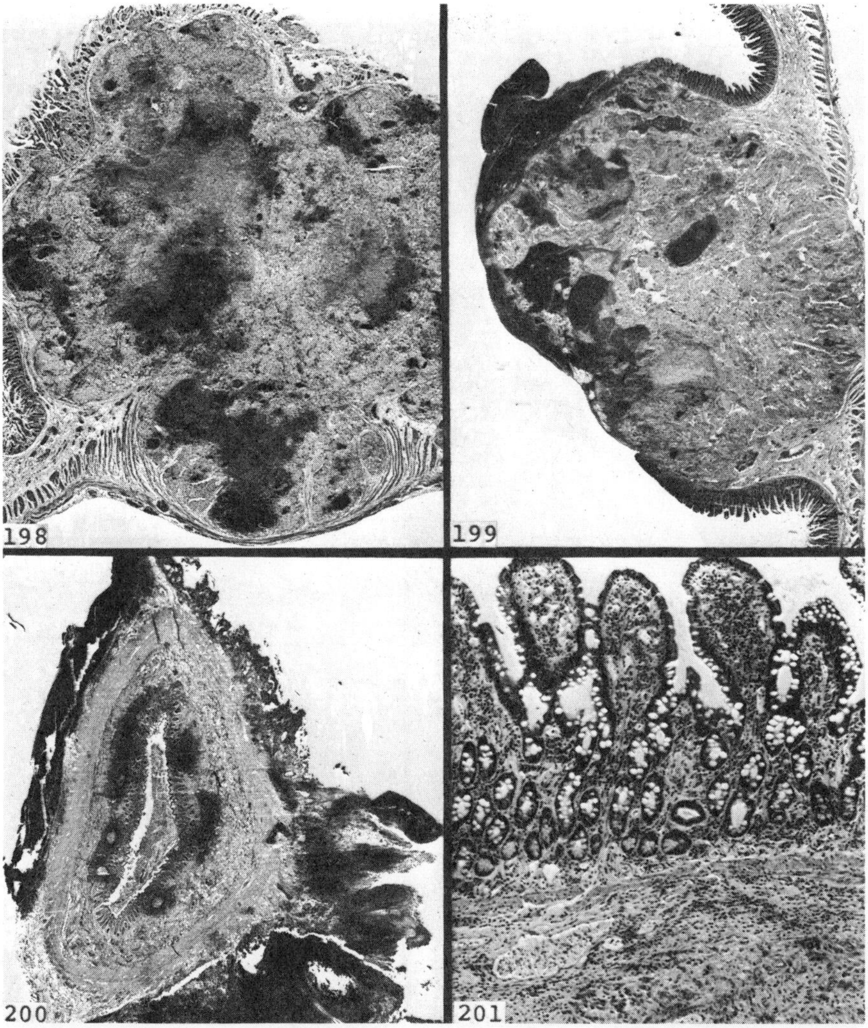

FIGURE 198. *Case 23:* Small intestine 15 months after a hydatidiform mole, showing a metastatic deposit of choriocarcinoma in the submucosa expanding centrifugally to produce superficial ulceration of the mucosa and pressure atrophy of the muscularis just short of perforating the serosa. (× 10)

FIGURE 199. *Case 36:* Small intestine 34 months after a spontaneous abortion, showing a nodule of metastatic choriocarcinoma in the submucosa which has produced ulceration and hemorrhage at the mucosal surface. (× 11)

FIGURE 200. *Case 9:* Vermiform appendix 8 months after term delivery. Choriocarcinoma perforating the uterus led to terminal hemoperitoneum; the appendix was adherent to the uterine mass, surrounded by blood clot, and shows a thin layer of trophoblast growing on its serosa (see FIGURE 18). (× 7)

FIGURE 201. *Case 33:* Small intestine resected at laparotomy 35 months after a hydatidiform mole, showing metastatic choriocarcinoma in the submucosa. The muscularis mucosae is preserved and the mucosa undisturbed. (× 60)

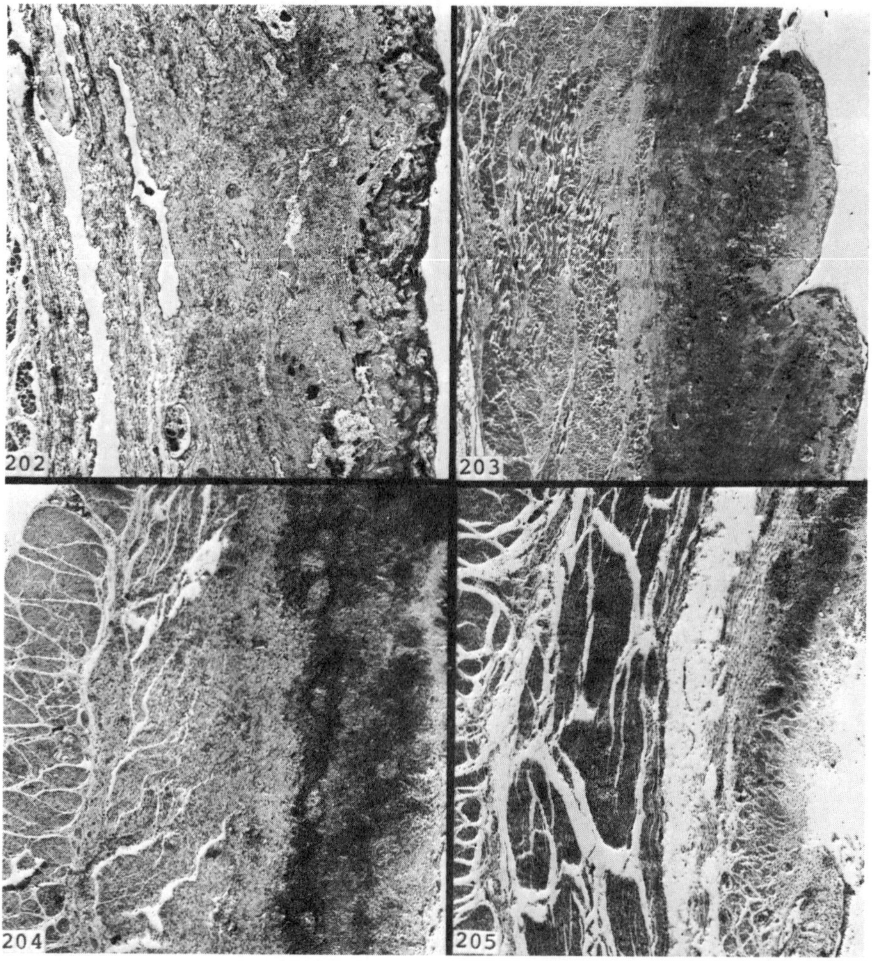

FIGURE 202. *Case 43:* Tongue 1 month after choriocarcinoma was diagnosed at craniotomy and treated with one course of methotrexate, showing necrotizing membranous glossitis. Bacterial colonies are seen on the surface and in underlying veins. (× 32)

FIGURE 203. *Case 43:* Esophagus from the same patient as in FIGURE 202, showing similar features. (× 11)

FIGURE 204. *Case 41:* Esophagus 14 months after a spontaneous abortion, followed by treatment of choriocarcinoma with several courses of oral methotrexate, then six courses of actinomycin-D, then methotrexate intramuscularly. The esophageal mucosa is destroyed and replaced by necrotic pseudomembrane. (× 23)

FIGURE 205. *Case 13:* Esophagus 2 years after term delivery, followed by nephrectomy, then five courses of methotrexate, five of actinomycin-D, and one of "triple therapy," showing acute ulceration of the mucosa and inflammatory exudate in the submucosa. (× 28)

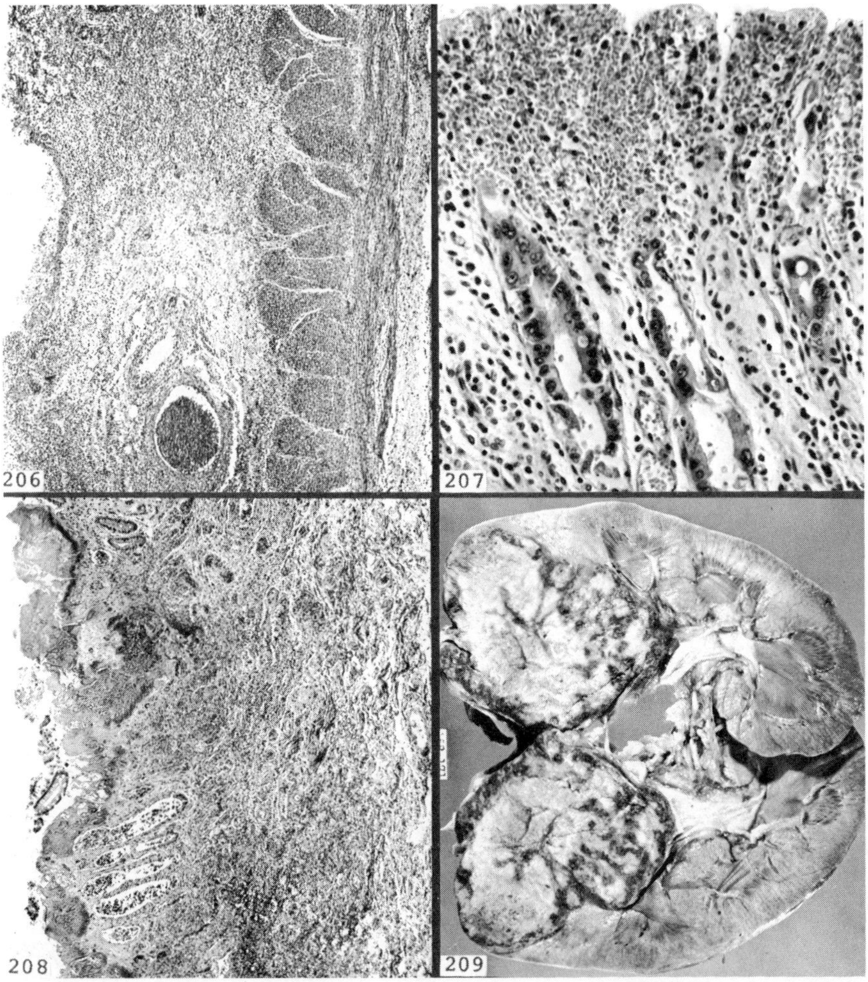

FIGURE 206. *Case 19:* Small intestine 22 months after a hydatidiform mole. Patient received six courses of methotrexate during the last 3 months of life. The mucosa is denuded of glandular elements, and a diffuse leukocytic exudate infiltrates the enteric wall through to the peritoneum. A submucosal vein is thrombosed. ($\times$ 36)

FIGURE 207. *Case 34:* Small intestine 40 months after a hydatidiform mole. During the last 6 months of life the patient received three courses of methotrexate, four of actinomycin-D, three of actinomycin-D with chlorambucil, and, preterminally, one of leukocristine. The mucosa is atrophic, showing atypical cells in remaining glands, and there is superficial hemorrhage. ($\times$ 144)

FIGURE 208. *Case 8:* Large intestine 11 months after term delivery, seven courses of methotrexate, and two of vincaleukoblastine, showing diffuse pseudomembranous colitis. ($\times$ 37)

FIGURE 209. *Case 1:* Kidney at autopsy 1 year after term delivery, showing a 7-cm, partially hemorrhagic, partially necrotic metastasis of choriocarcinoma in the lower pole.

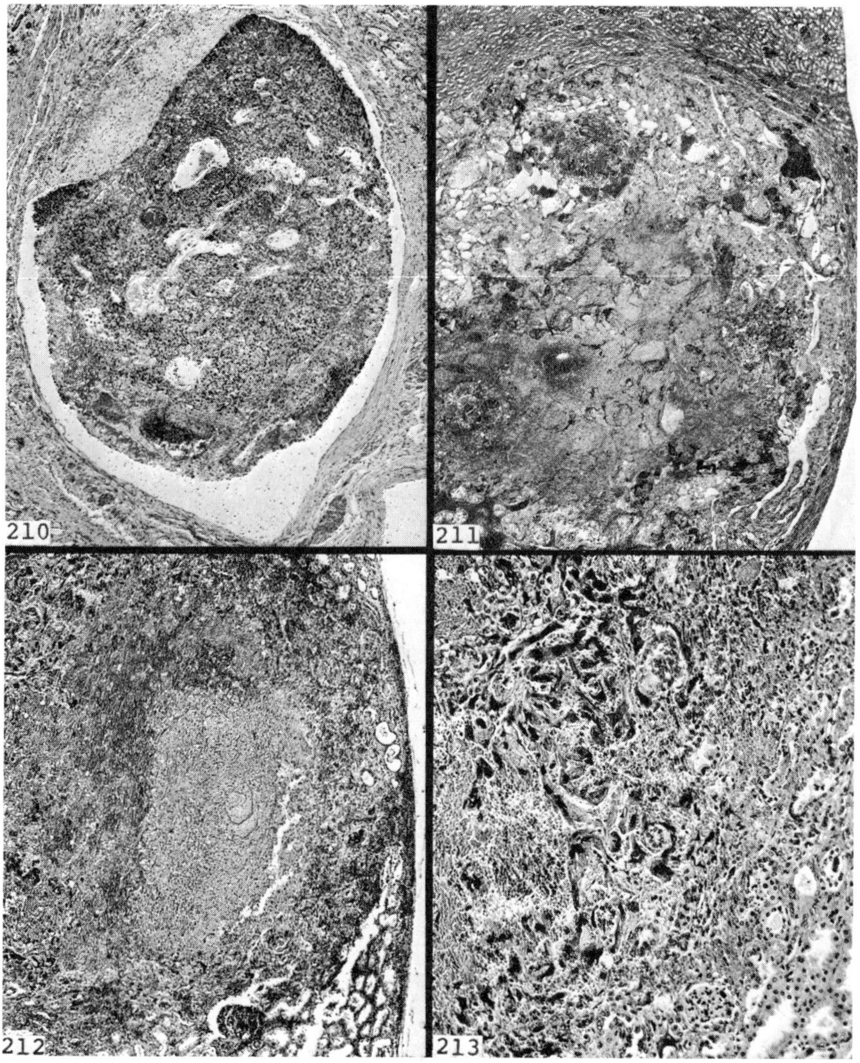

FIGURE 210. *Case 30:* Kidney at autopsy 46 months after a hydatidiform mole, showing a large embolus of choriocarcinoma attached to the wall of an intrarenal vein. (× 32)

FIGURE 211. *Case 10:* Kidney 20.5 months after term delivery, showing a nodule of metastatic choriocarcinoma in the cortex, with central hemorrhage and necrosis. (× 12)

FIGURE 212. *Case 3:* Kidney 10 months after term delivery, showing a nodule of metastatic choriocarcinoma in the cortex, with central necrosis. (× 35)

FIGURE 213. *Case 3:* Detail from the margin of FIGURE 212, showing neoplastic trophoblast infiltrating between tubules in the cortex. (× 86)

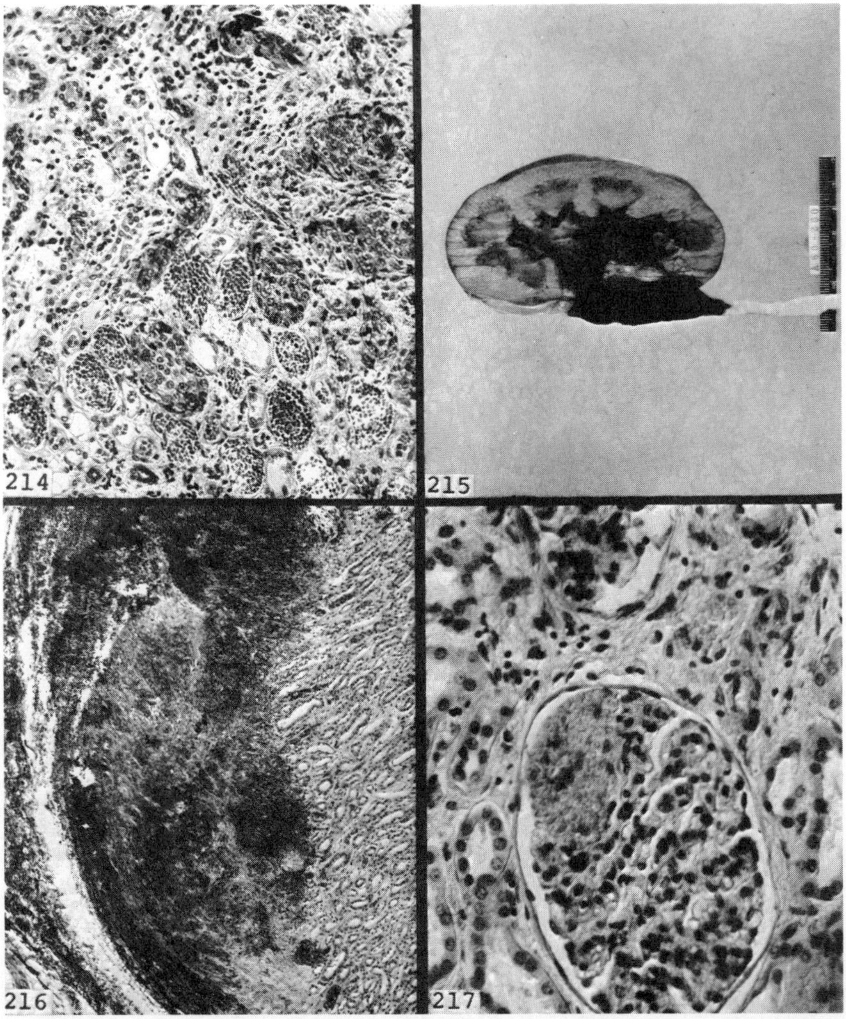

FIGURE 214. *Case 26:* Kidney 35 months after a hydatidiform mole, showing nests of metastatic choriocarcinoma disrupting the tubular architecuture. (× 132)

FIGURE 215. *Case 8:* Kidney at autopsy 11 months after term delivery, showing extensive hemorrhage in the renal pelvis and ureter. After seven courses of methotrexate and two of vincaleukoblastine, pancytopenia developed. The bone marrow was hypoplastic, and hemorrhagic phenomena were found elsewhere.

FIGURE 216. *Case 8:* Kidney showing fresh hemorrhage into renal pelvis at the tip of a pyramid. (× 42)

FIGURE 217. *Case 22:* Kidney 28 months after a hydatidiform mole. Patient received five courses of methotrexate during the last months of life. Segmental necrosis of the glomeruli is interpreted as a possible toxic effect of medication. (×216)

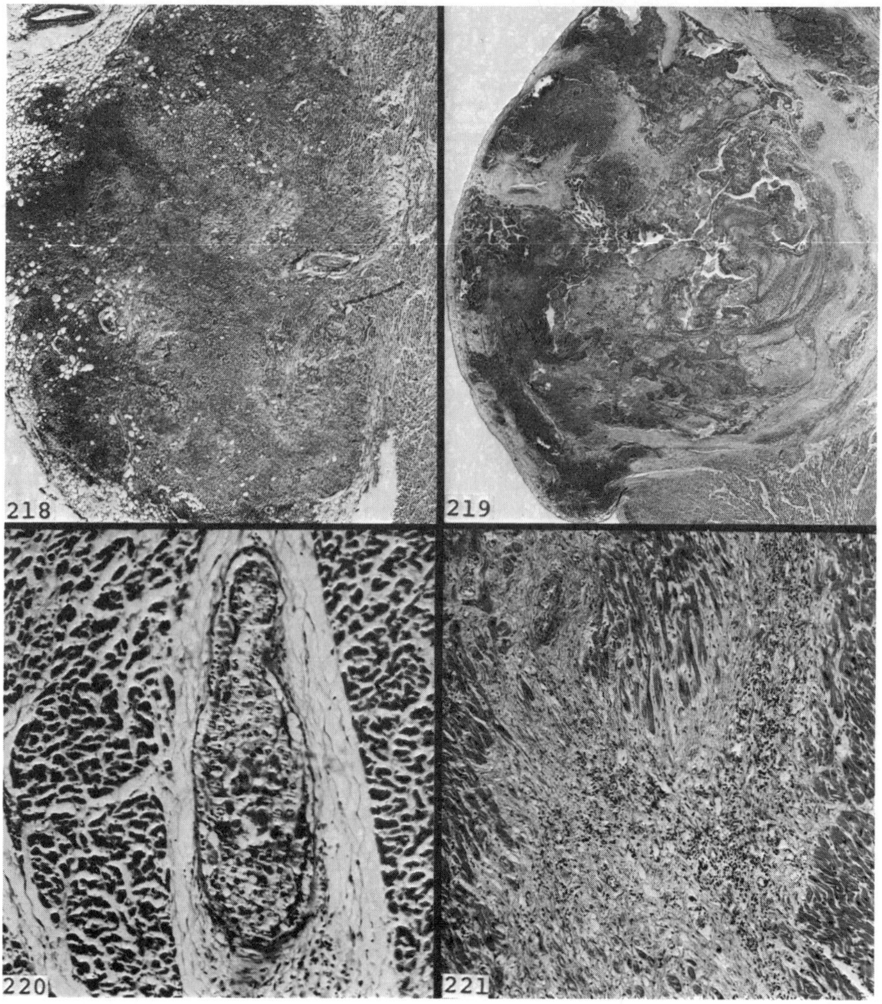

FIGURE 218. *Case 1:* Heart 1 year after term delivery, showing a nodule of metastatic choriocarcinoma in the epicardial fat. (× 9)

FIGURE 219. *Case 11:* Heart 10 months after term delivery, showing a largely necrotic nodule of metastatic choriocarcinoma in the wall of the left ventricle, projecting as a boss on the epicardial surface. (× 11)

FIGURE 220. *Case 4:* Heart 8 months after delivery in an untreated patient, showing a small embolic mass of trophoblast occluding a small branch of the coronary artery tree. (× 80)

FIGURE 221. *Case 4:* An adjacent field on the same slide shown in FIGURE 220, showing a small focus of healing myocardial infarction. (× 60)

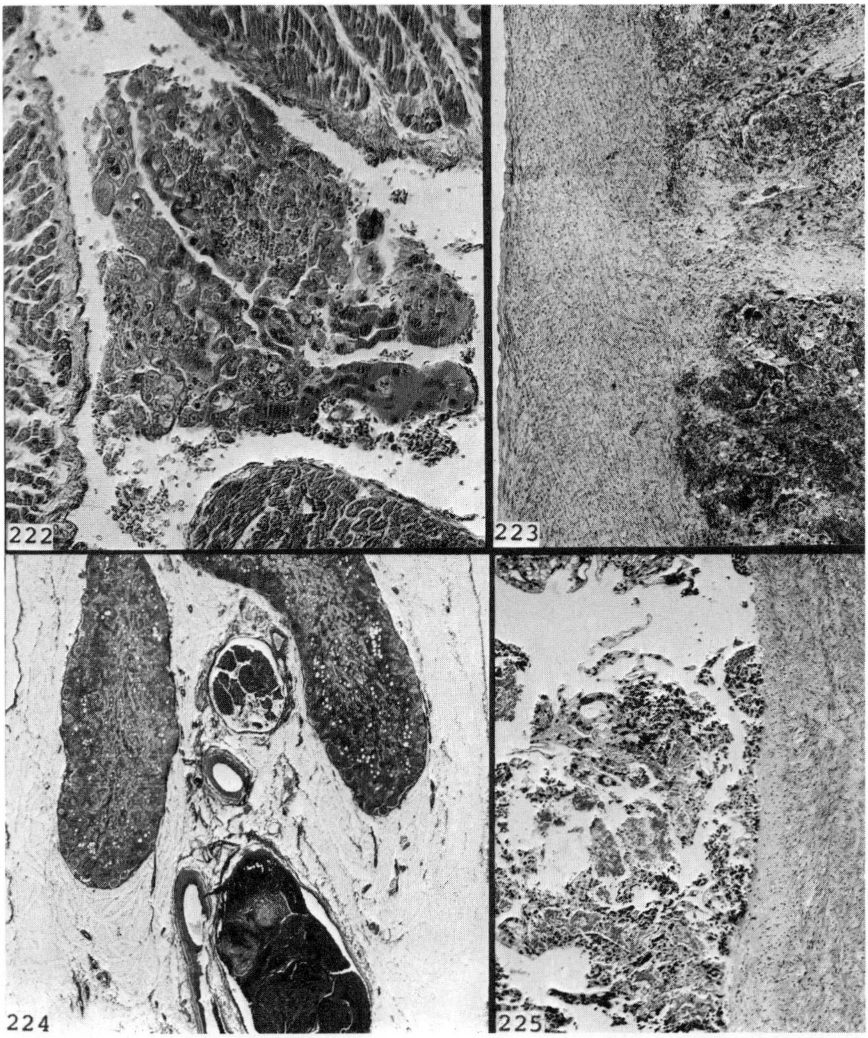

FIGURE 222. *Case 21:* Heart 5 months after a hydatidiform mole, showing a nest of embolic trophoblast trapped in a recess of the trabeculae carnae of the right ventricle. (× 112)

FIGURE 223. *Case 15:* Aorta 1 year postpartum, showing metastatic choriocarcinoma in the adventitia but not invading the media. (× 30)

FIGURE 224. *Case 27:* Full thickness of mesentery in patient dying 26 months after a hydatidiform mole. Extensive metastases of choriocarcinoma were found in intra-abdominal organs, including the pancreas (see FIGURE 188). There is terminal thrombosis of a ramus of the mesenteric venous drainage. (× 4)

FIGURE 225. *Case 30:* Main left branch of the pulmonary artery 46 months after a hydatidiform mole, showing a portion of the mass of neoplastic trophoblast attached to the intima and partially obstructing the lumen. (× 35)

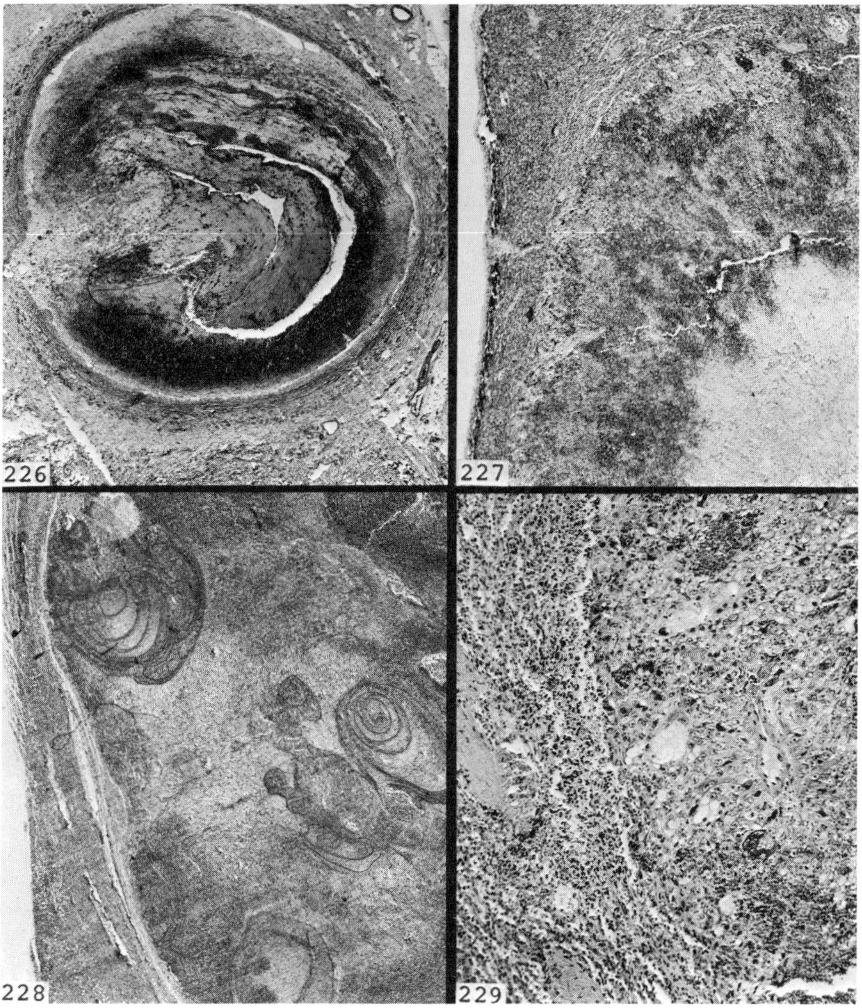

FIGURE 226. *Case 10:* Pelvic vessels 20.5 months after term delivery, showing phlebothrombosis not associated with nearby tumor. (× 12)

FIGURE 227. *Case 5:* Nodule in a spleen 7 months postpartum, showing viable trophoblast at the periphery of a zone of hemorrhage surrounding a central zone of coagulation necrosis. (× 18)

FIGURE 228. *Case 5:* Spleen 7 months postpartum, showing a large hemorrhagic nodule without viable trophoblast in the field. (× 12)

FIGURE 229. *Case 25:* Spleen 28 months after a hydatidiform mole, showing metastatic choriocarcinoma abutting the red pulp. (× 67)

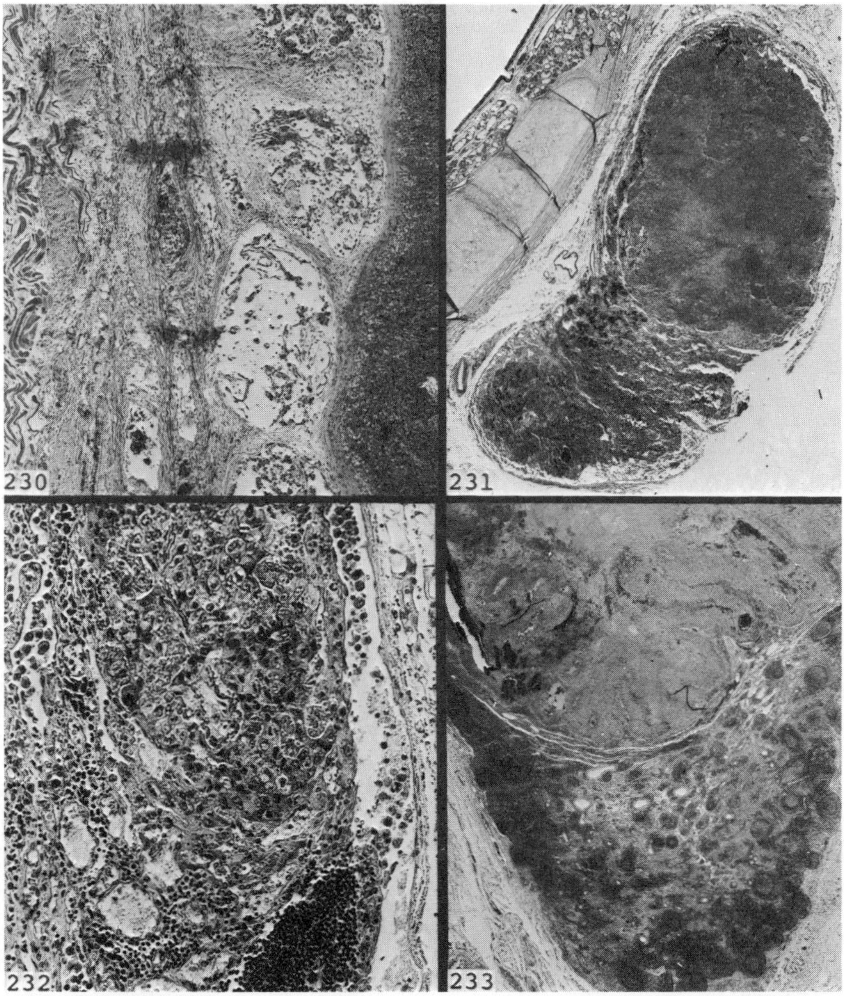

FIGURE 230. *Case 54:* Spleen and diaphram 10 weeks after resection of an ovarian tumor containing both disgerminoma and choriocarcinoma, showing clusters of neoplastic trophoblast permeating veins in fibrous tissue that has created lienophrenic adhesion (× 28)

FIGURE 231. *Case 1:* Paratracheal lymph node 1 year after term delivery in a patient dying with extensive secondary pulmonary deposits of choriocarcinoma (see FIGURES 149 & 150). A portion of the node is replaced by a necrotic tertiary deposit. (× 10)

FIGURE 232. *Case 1:* Omental lymph node, showing a small deposit of choriocarcinoma beneath the marginal sinus. The patient had a solitary metastasis to the stomach (see FIGURE 194). The cortex of the node is depleted of lymphoid cells as a result of chemotherapy. (× 108)

FIGURE 233. *Case 33:* Mesenteric lymph node draining a segment of the small intestine with a secondary deposit of choriocarcinoma 35 months after a hydatidiform mole. The node contains a necrotic tertiary deposit of choriocarcinoma (see FIGURE 201). (× 7)

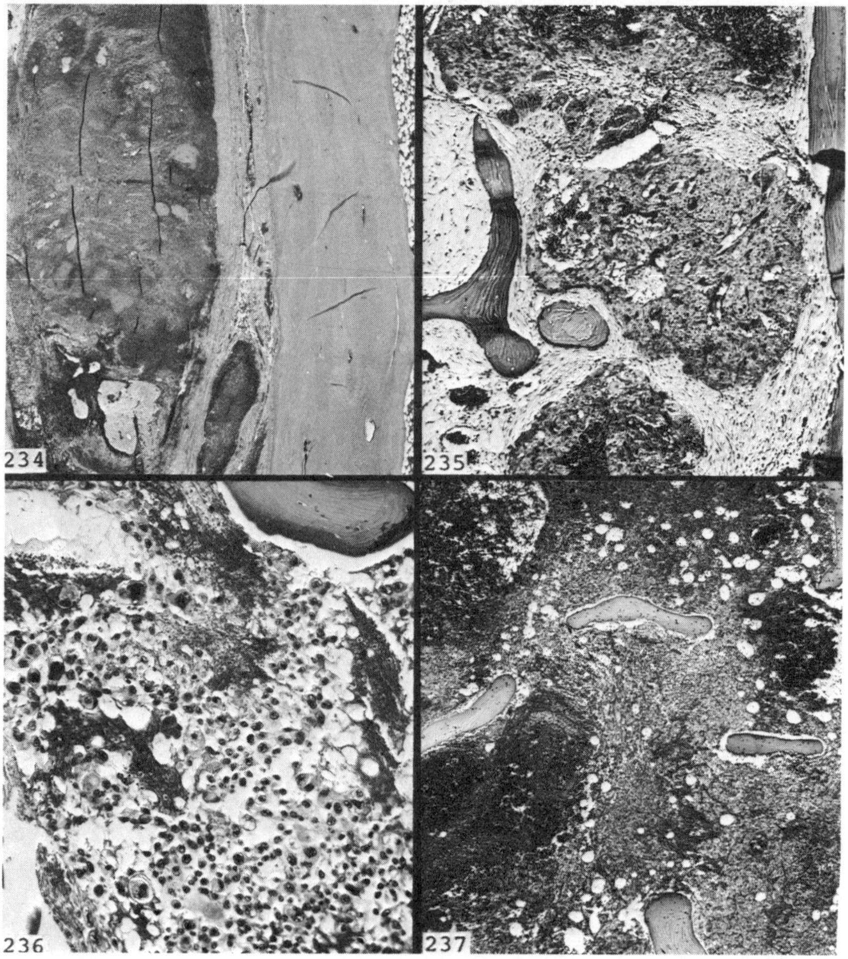

FIGURE 234. *Case 39:* Rib at autopsy 14 months after a spontaneous abortion, showing a nodule of choriocarcinoma metastatic to the periosteum. (× 11)

FIGURE 235. *Case 20:* Vertebral body 23 months after a hydatidiform mole, showing nests of metastatic choriocarcinoma near cortical bone. Despite five courses of methotrexate, two of vincaleukoblastine, and other chemotherapy, only the marrow adjacent to metastatic tumor is depleted of cells; the marrow elsewhere was normal. Local marrow depletion is interpreted as the result of competition for folate by tumor cells against nearby marrow cells. (× 47)

FIGURE 236. *Case 38:* Bone marrow from lumbar vertebra 10 months after a spontaneous abortion in an untreated patient, showing metastatic choriocarcinoma destroying bone. (× 75)

FIGURE 237. *Case 35:* Bone marrow 23 months after a hydatidiform mole. Following five courses of methotrexate, three of actinomycin-D, and four of "triple therapy," pancytopenia developed. Much of the marrow is overrun by old and recent hemorrhage. (× 30)

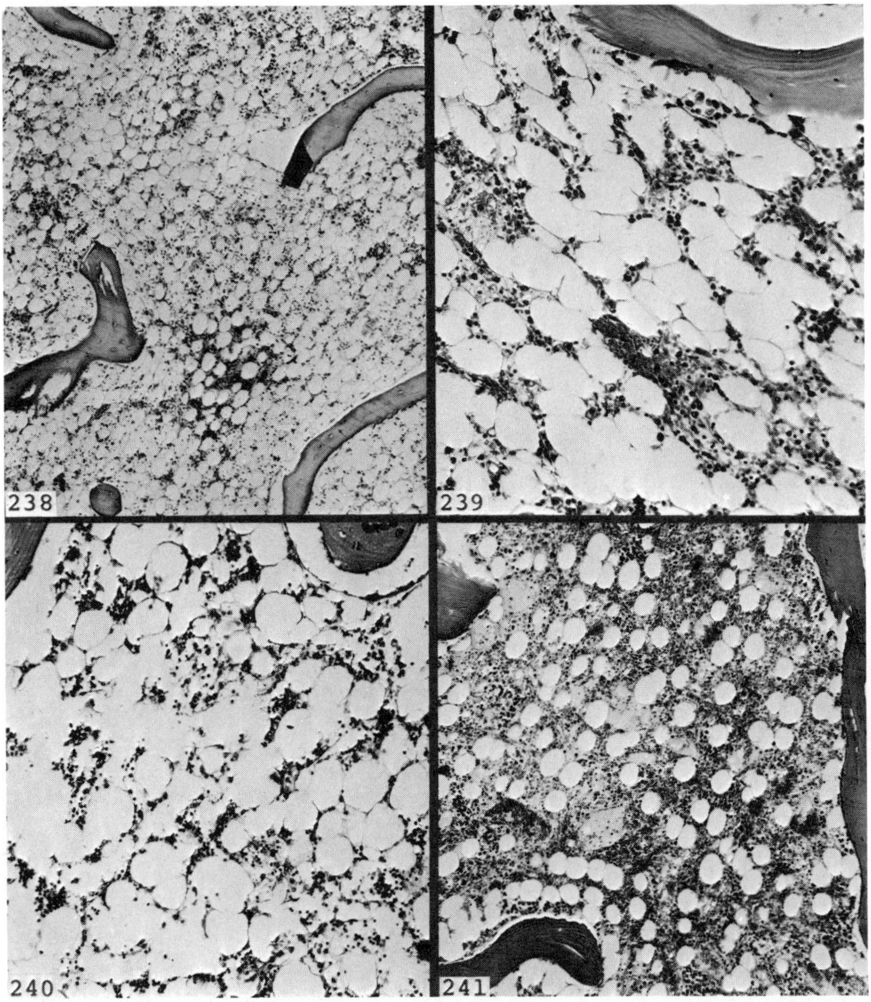

FIGURE 238. *Case 41:* Bone marrow 14 months after an abortion. The patient received several courses of oral methotrexate and six of actinomycin-D, as well as methotrexate intramuscularly preterminally. There is severe depletion of erythropoietic, myelopoietic, and thrombocytopoietic elements. (see FIGURE 204). (× 76)

FIGURE 239. *Case 22:* Bone marrow 28 months after a hydatidiform mole. The patient received five courses of methotrexate during the last 8 months of life. The marrow shows depletion of all cellular elements; megakaryocytes are almost entirely absent. (× 76)

FIGURE 240. *Case 43:* Bone marrow 1 month after choriocarcinoma was diagnosed at craniotomy. The patient received one course of methotrexate. There is almost complete destruction of erythropoietic and myelopoietic cells; megakaryocytes are absent (see FIGURE 202). (× 100)

FIGURE 241. *Case 8:* Bone marrow 11 months after term delivery. The patient received seven courses of methotrexate and two of vincaleukoblastine. Although the marrow seems to show a relatively normal cell-to-fat ratio, cellular depletion is present (× 52)

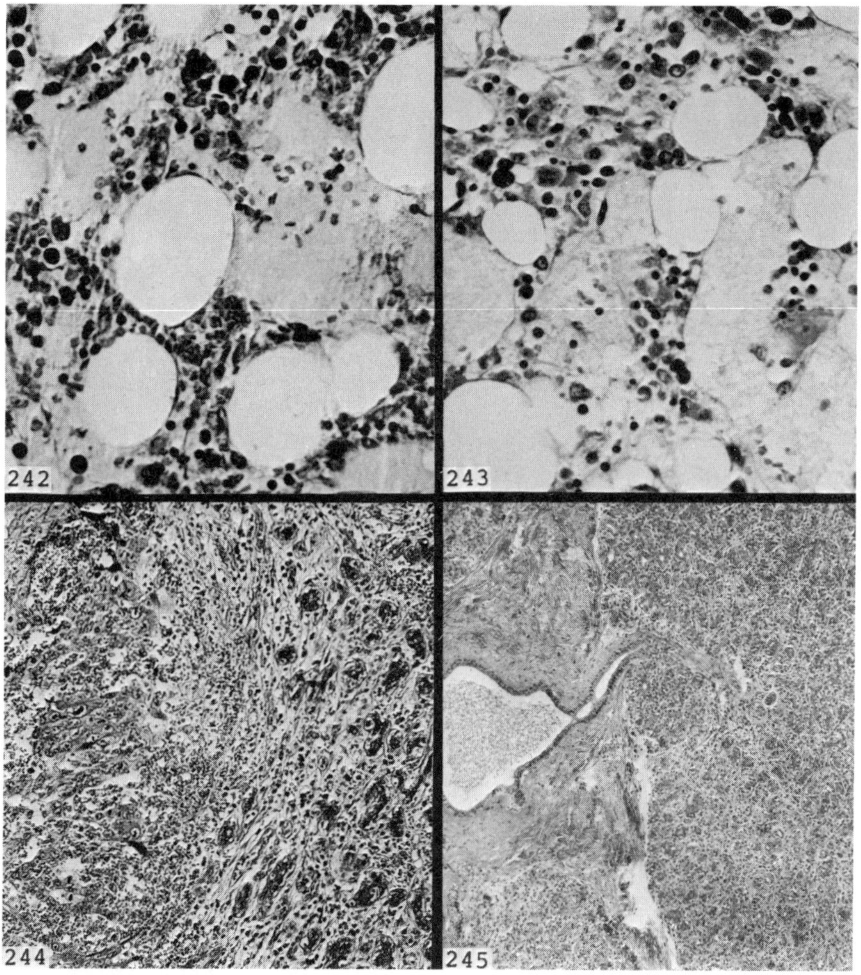

FIGURE 242. *Case 8:* Detail of FIGURE 241, showing that the apparent cellularity is due to extravasation of erythrocytes between fat cells. Myeloid elements are degenerated and destroyed; there is granular alteration of the cytoplasm of fat cells (see FIGURES 208 & 215). (× 232)

FIGURE 243. *Case 34:* Bone marrow 40 months after a hydatidiform mole. The patient received three courses of methotrexate, four of actinomycin-D, three of actinomycin-D and chlorambucil, and one of leukocristine. Almost all cellular elements have disappeared from the marrow, and there is degeneration of the few remaining cells. The marrow fat cells contain granular material (see FIGURES 184, 193, & 207). (× 208)

FIGURE 244. *Case 2:* Section of a mass in a breast excised 18 months postpartum, showing choriocarcinoma infiltrating hyperplastic lobular tissue. The neoplasm is extremely hemorrhagic; lobular hyperplasia was not prominent away from the tumor. (× 86)

FIGURE 245. *Case 4:* Breast at autopsy 8 months after term delivery showing a hyperplastic lobule and a dilated duct containing products of secretion. (× 52)

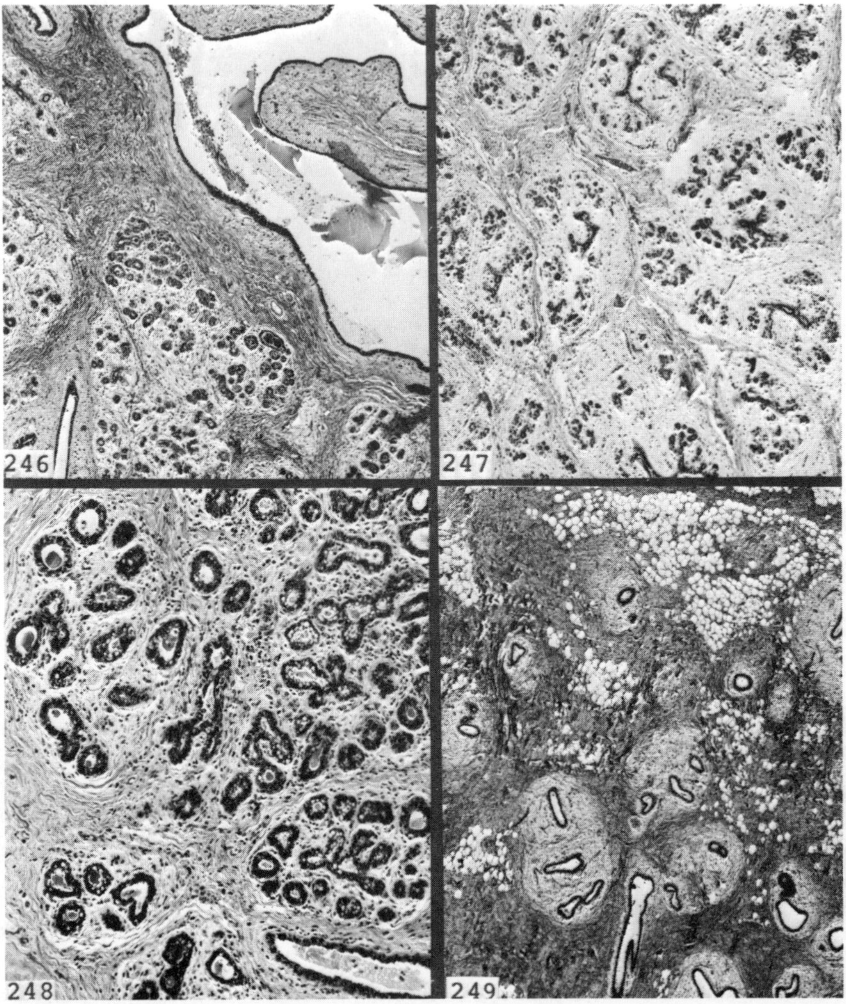

FIGURE 246. *Case 20:* Breast at autopsy 23 months after a hydatidiform mole, showing hyperplasia of intrinsic lobular stroma and a dilated major duct containing products of gland secretion. (× 32)

FIGURE 247. *Case 30:* Breast at autopsy 46 months after a hydatidiform mole, showing pronounced lobular hyperplasia due chiefly to an increase in intrinsic lobular stroma. (× 30)

FIGURE 248. *Case 28:* Breast at autopsy 10 months after a hydatidiform mole, showing moderate hyperplasia of a terminal lobule. Secretory vacuolation of the glandular epithelium and intraluminal secretion are present. (× 71)

FIGURE 249. *Case 53:* Breast at autopsy of a 9-year-old girl, 13 months after resection of ovarian teratocarcinoma with choriocarcinoma, showing dilated ducts and hyperplasia of periductal stroma but no development of lobules. (× 16)

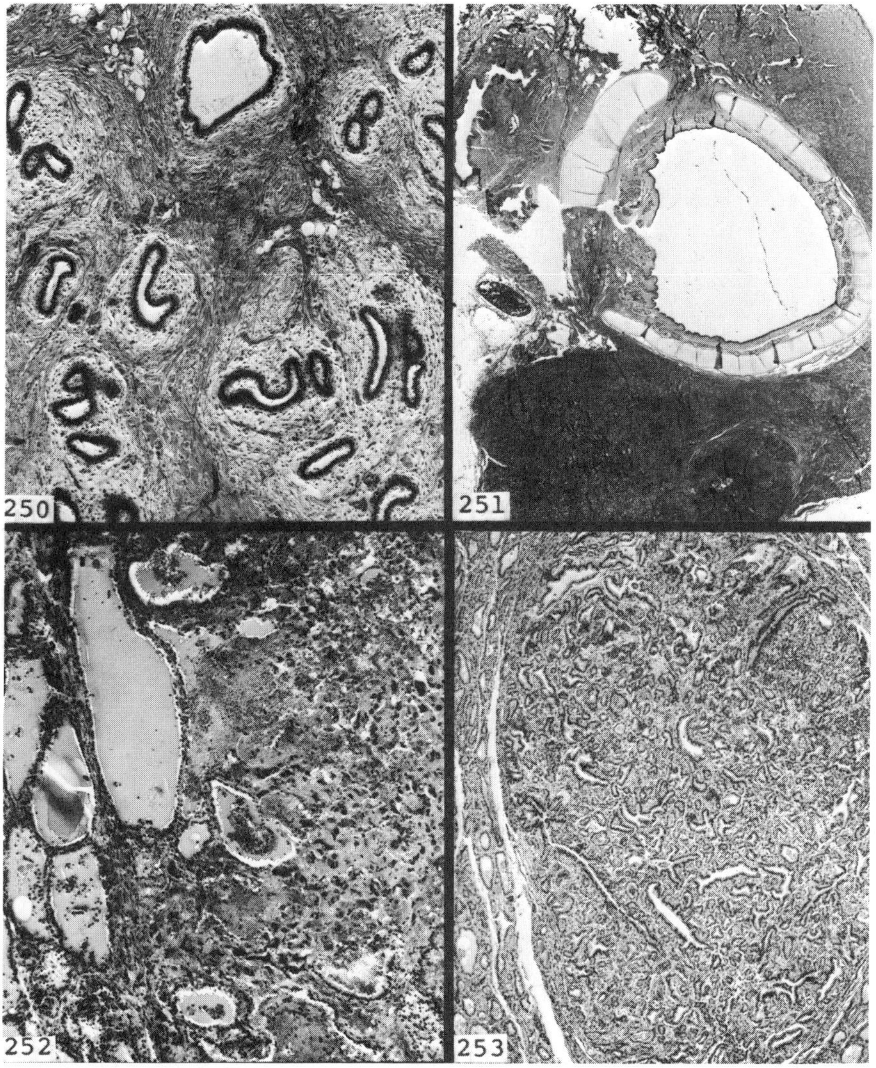

FIGURE 250. *Case 53:* Detail of FIGURE 249, showing similarity to gynecomastia in the male breast. (× 43)

FIGURE 251. *Case 4:* Cross-section of neck organs at autopsy 8 months postpartum, showing a discrete nodule of somewhat hemorrhagic choriocarcinoma in the right lobe of the thyroid gland. (× 3)

FIGURE 252. *Case 3:* Thyroid gland at autopsy 10 months after term delivery, showing metastatic choriocarcinoma destroying thyroid follicles. (× 55)

FIGURE 253. *Case 19:* Thyroid gland at autopsy 22 months after a hydatidiform mole, showing focal follicular hyperplasia. Intercurrent hyperthyroidism developed during treatment and was managed by methimazole. (× 41)

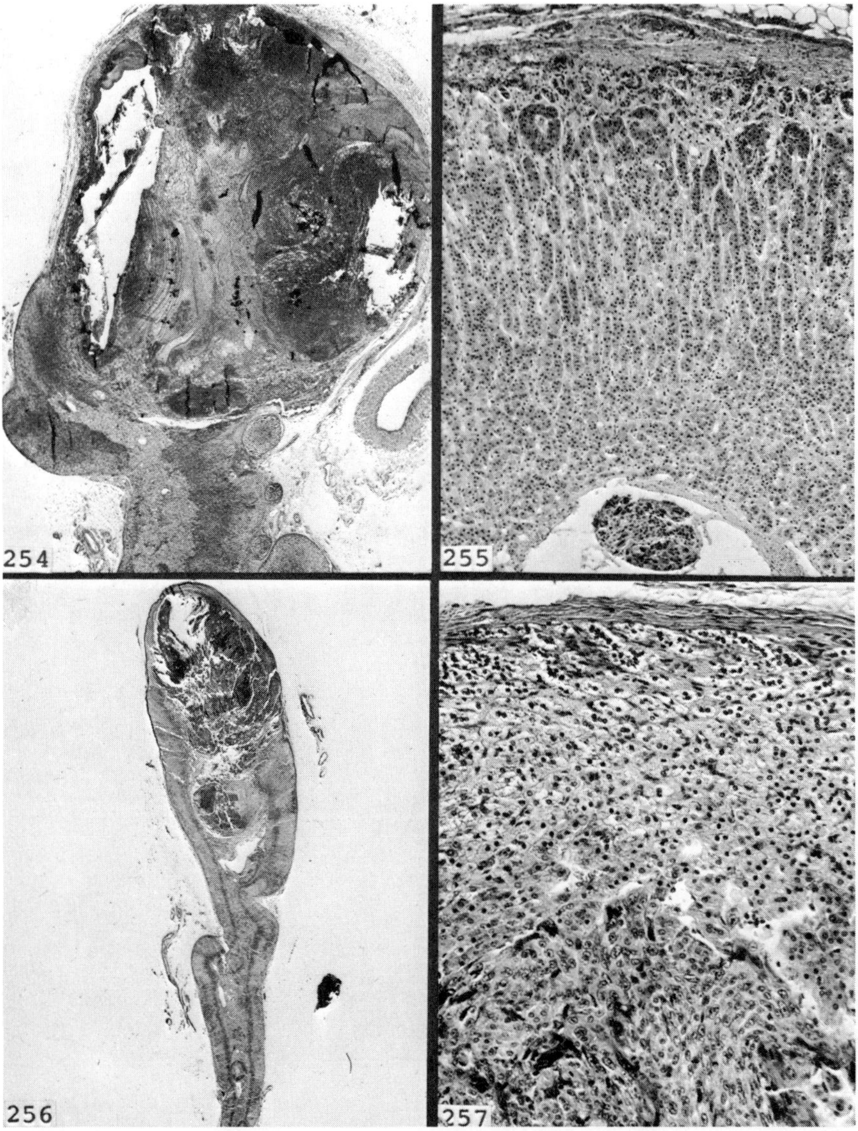

FIGURE 254. *Case 40:* Adrenal gland 11 months after a spontaneous abortion, showing a relatively large hemorrhagic nodule of choriocarcinoma at one pole. (× 7)

FIGURE 255. *Case 29:* Adrenal gland at autopsy 4 years after a hydatidiform mole, showing an embolus of choriocarcinoma in the central vein. (× 55)

FIGURE 256. *Case 26:* Adrenal gland 35 months after a hyaditiform mole, showing metastatic choriocarcinoma in the medulla, impinging on the cortex. (× 3.4)

FIGURE 257. Detail of FIGURE 256, showing sheets of neoplastic trophoblast infiltrating cortex. (× 115)

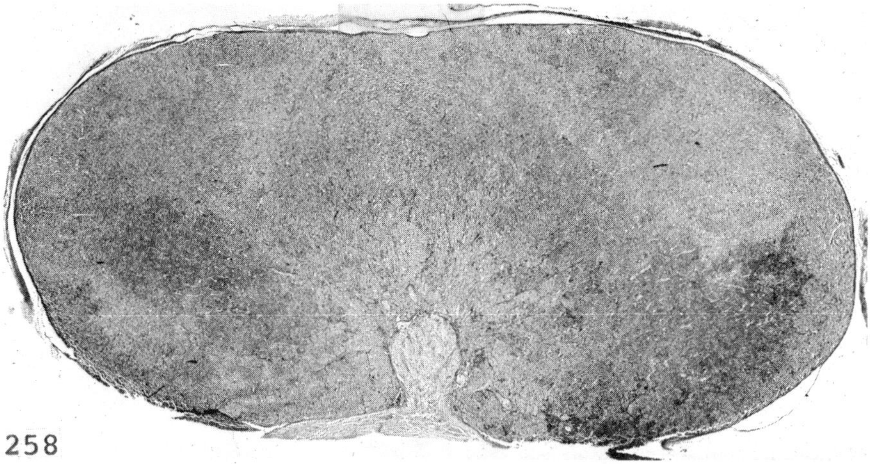

258

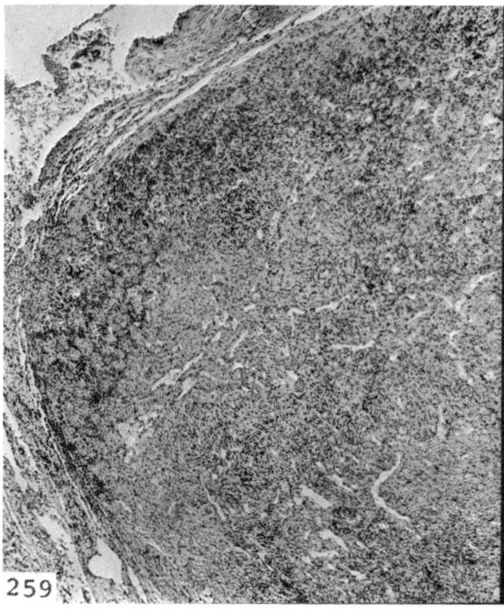

259

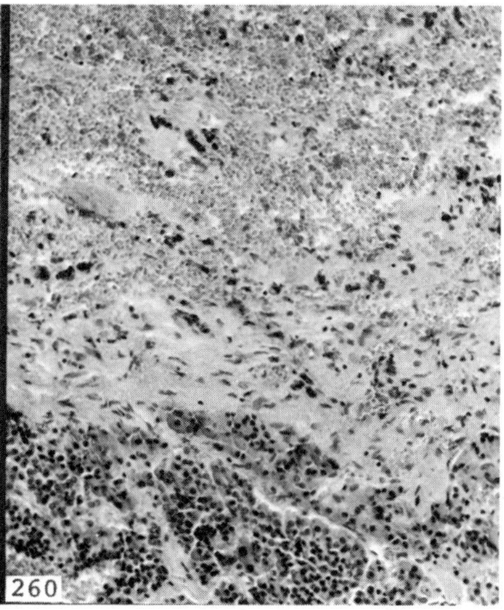

260

FIGURE 258. *Case 38:* Crosssection of the anterior pituitary gland 10 months after a spontaneous abortion, showing patchy areas of necrosis. (× 7)

FIGURE 259. *Case 25:* Pituitary gland 28 months after a hydatidiform mole, showing coagulation necrosis of the anterior lobe, with light leukocytic infiltration. A few viable cells remain beneath the capsule. (× 60)

FIGURE 260. *Case 25:* Detail of FIGURE 259, showing viable pituitary cells between the zone of necrosis and the capsule. (× 120)

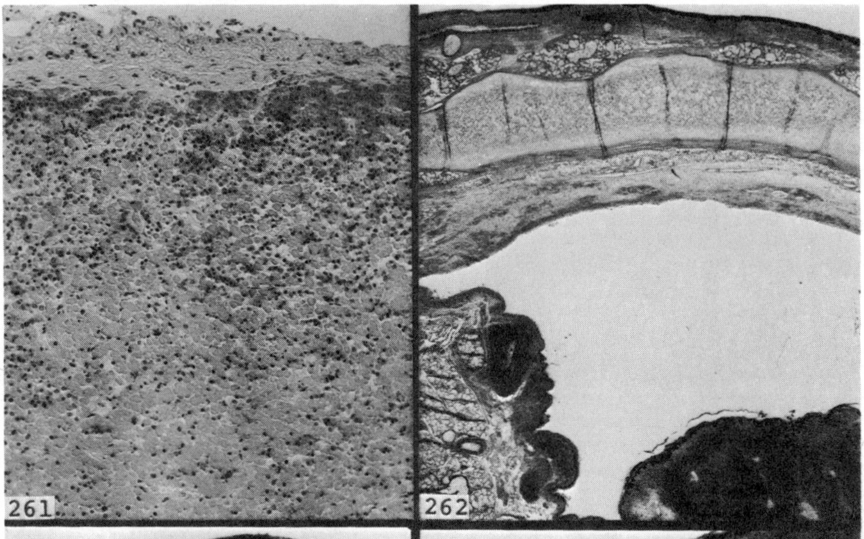

FIGURE 261. *Case 29:* Pituitary gland 4 years after a hydatidiform mole, showing necrosis involving most of a lateral lobe. (× 16)

FIGURE 262. *Case 41:* Epiglottis and adjacent hypopharynx 14 months after a spontaneous abortion. The patient received six courses of antinomycin-D and at least one course of methotrexate. The mucosa on the posterior surface and tip are denuded of epithelium and bacterial colonies are growing on the denuded surface. (× 11)

FIGURE 263. *Case 41:* Detail from a field adjacent to that shown in 262, showing the denuded surface and bacterial colonies (see FIGURE 238). (× 60)

FIGURE 264. *Case 8:* Epiglottis 11 months after term delivery. The patient received seven courses of methotrexate and two of vincaleukoblastine. The mucosa is destroyed; there is necrosis in the submucosa and thrombosis of a submucosal vein (see FIGURE 241). (× 35)

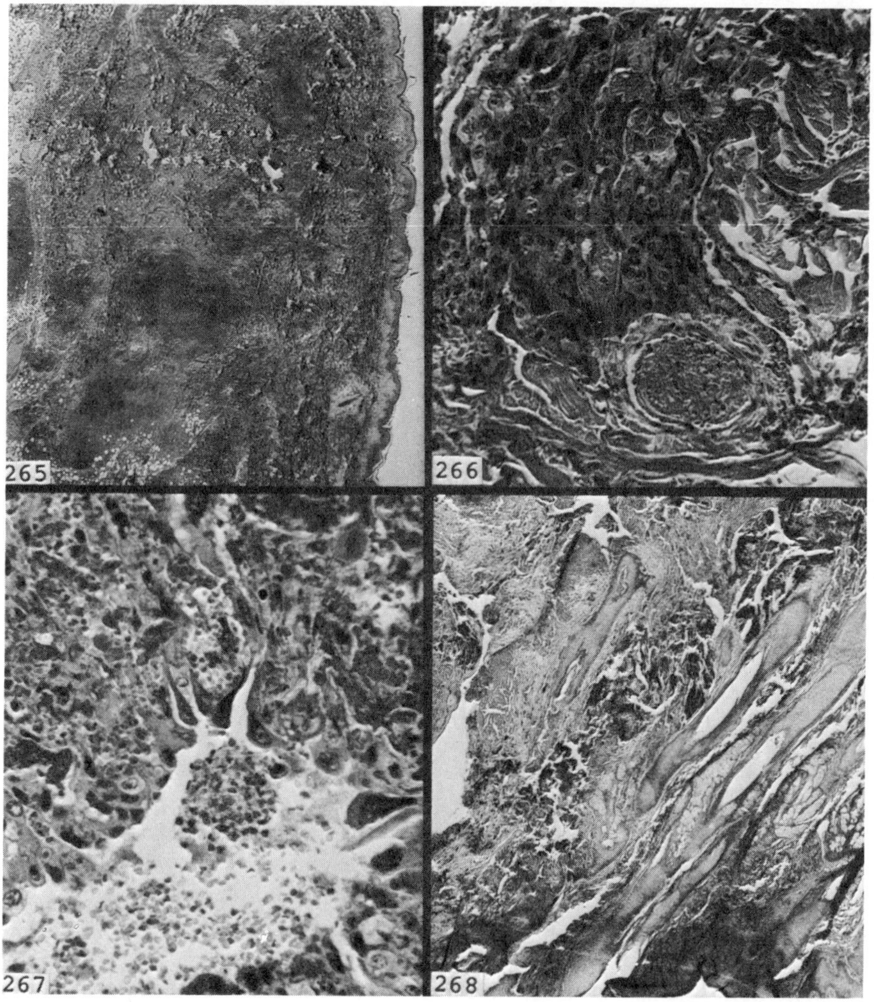

FIGURE 265. *Case 35:* Skin from a shoulder at autopsy 23 months after a hydatidiform mole, showing an ill-defined hemorrhagic lesion in the dermis. (× 16)

FIGURE 266. *Case 35:* Detail of FIGURE 265, showing a clump of neoplastic trophoblast in the corium near a peripheral nerve fiber. (× 160)

FIGURE 267. *Case 35:* Detail of FIGURE 265, showing neoplastic trophoblast surrounding a blood-filled space. (× 232)

FIGURE 268. *Case 87:* Nodule excised from scalp 8.5 months after a spontaneous abortion, showing sheets of neoplastic trophoblast infiltrating corium and between hair shifts. (× 18)

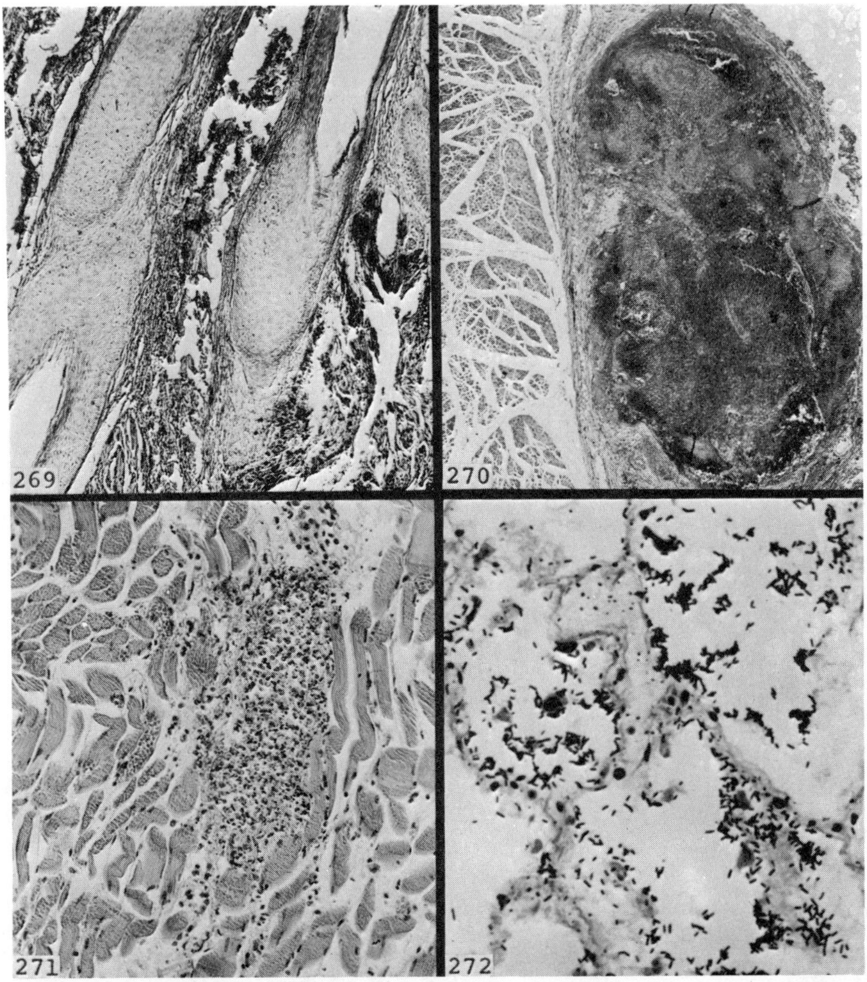

FIGURE 269. *Case 87:* Detail of FIGURE 268, showing cellular components of choriocarcinoma. The patient was reported living and well 7 years after discharge. (× 52)

FIGURE 270. *Case 5:* Right gastrocnemius muscle 7 months after term delivery, showing a hemorrhagic deposit of choriocarcinoma in its fascial sheath. (× 13)

FIGURE 271. *Case 22:* Psoas muscle from a patient dying with pancytopenia and peritonitis, 28 months after a hydatidiform mole treated with five courses of methotrexate, showing a microabscess secondary to disseminated terminal sepsis (see FIGURE 239). (× 112)

FIGURE 272. *Case 54:* Lung 10 weeks after removal of an ovarian tumor composed of disgerminoma and choriocarcinoma, showing a large number of gram-positive bacilli identified in culture as *Clostridium perfringens.* (× 232)

Appendix: Epitome of Cases of Choriocarcinoma

GROUP I: Fatal Cases of Gestational Choriocarcinoma, Autopsied

Following Term Delivery

Case 1: L.B. (00–83–92), a 26-year-old gravida 2, para 2, had her second term delivery in July, 1957. About 3 months later she developed headache, weakness, nausea, vomiting, and paresis of the left arm, followed by visual-field disturbance. Electroencephalography revealed a space-occupying lesion in the posterior part of the right cerebral hemisphere, and craniotomy in February, 1958, 7 months postpartum, revealed a metastatic choriocaricinoma. A chest x-ray showed multiple nodules in both lungs, and she was admitted to NIH on February 28, 1958. The HCG titer on admission was 1 million units, and then declined to about 100,000 units after five courses of methotrexate over the next 2 months. Symptoms referable to the central nervous system increased in May, 1958, and she was treated with methotrexate intravenously and intrathecally, and then with 2-deoxyglucose. Hypophysectomy was performed on June 18, but she died on July 29, 1958, 5 months after admission and 1 year after delivery.

Autopsy (A-58–171) revealed choriocarcinoma metastatic to the brain, lungs (FIGURES 149–151), liver, kidneys (FIGURE 209), stomach (FIGURE 194), peritoneum, heart (FIGURE 218), left submaxillary gland, and mediastinal and omental lymph nodes (FIGURES 231 & 232). There was no choriocarcinoma in the uterus, but the endometrium showed a weak decidual reaction (FIGURES 73 & 74). A few small theca-lutein cysts were present in the ovaries (FIGURE 104), and also an ectopic decidual reaction (FIGURE 116). There was no substantive evidence of remission of this patient's disease, and she died of widely disseminated choriocarcinoma.

Case 2: R.B. (01–78–42), a 39-year-old gravida 3, para 3, had her third term delivery in February, 1956, a cesarean section followed by tubal ligation. Menses resumed cyclically, and she was in good health until May, 1957, some 15 months later, when vaginal spotting appeared. On May 27, 1957, she had an episode of severe hemoptysis followed by shock, requiring hospitalization. A chest x-ray showed a large mass in the left lower lobe, and lobectomy on June 7, 1957, revealed this mass to be a metastatic choriocarcinoma. She was admitted to NIH on June 17, 1957; a chest x-ray revealed a few small nodules in both lung fields, and the HCG titer was 20,000 units. She was treated with seven courses of methotrexate, and the titer gradually fell to the level of 500–1,000 units. A mass developed in one breast during the early days of treatment; it was excised on July 22, 1957, and pathological examination revealed metastatic choriocarcinoma abutting secreting breast tissue (S-57–1098) (FIGURE 244). Under therapy, the chest nodules disappeared. The patient was discharged to the care of her referring physician on October 25, 1957. She remained well, with low HCG titers, until April 1, 1958, when she was admitted to a local hospital with the sudden onset of convulsion followed by coma. She died 3 hours after admission.

Autopsy* (A-58–81 revealed massive intracerebral hemorrhage secondary to metastatic choriocarcinoma (FIGURE 178). There was no other focus of choriocarcinoma in the body.

Case 3: M.D. (01–89–66), a 27-year-old gravida 2, para 1, aborta 1, had a term delivery in May, 1957. In July, 1957, 8 weeks postpartum, she developed persistent vaginal spotting, and 1 month later pain in the left lumbar region following a so-called respiratory infection. After the respiratory infection cleared, tinnitus developed. A chest x-ray showed bilateral pulmonary nodules consistent with metastatic disease, and a frog test was positive. Endometrial aspiration showed only decidual tissue. Signs of central nervous system involvement developed, and she was given a course of methotrexate therapy before being admitted to NIH on September 6, 1957, 4 months postpartum. The HCG titer on admission was 80,000 units, and a chest x-ray showed some decrease in the size of pulmonary nodules compared with the film taken prior to preadmission treatment. At NIH, she received four courses of methotrexate over 2 months, with a fall in the HCG titer to 10,000 units by November, 1957, and further reduction in the size of pulmonary nodules. However, no subsequent im-

*Autopsy performed by C. Merril Whorton, M.D., Jacksonville, Fla. (A-58–47).

provement was noted; despite intravenous methotrexate and further courses of oral methotrexate, the HCG titer rose progressively to the range of 16–20 million units, never declining below 4 million units, and new pulmonary lesions were demonstrated by repeated chest x-ray examinations. She died on March 17, 1958, 10 months postpartum and 6 months after admission.

Autopsy (A-58–61) revealed choriocarcinoma metastatic to the lungs (FIGURE 163), liver, jejunum (FIGURE 196), kidney (FIGURES 212 & 213), and thyroid gland (FIGURE 252). The immediate cause of death was massive gastrointestinal hemorrhage from the jejunal metastasis; there was also terminal bleeding in the lungs and liver. The ovaries exhibited a corpus luteum with calcospherites (FIGURE 111) and an ectopic pseudodecidual reaction (FIGURES 102 & 114); the endometrium showed diffuse decidual transformation. Lobular hyperplasia of the breasts was present.

Case 4: W.J. (01–04–07), a 39-year-old gravida 7, para 7, had her last term delivery on December 25, 1954. Continuous vaginal bleeding followed, and 1 month postpartum a "sore" appeared on the vaginal mucosa. A second vaginal lesion appeared 3 weeks later, and a biopsy was diagnosed as choriocarcinoma. Abdominal hysterectomy was performed 1 week later, 8 weeks postpartum, but vaginal bleeding continued as a hemorrhagic mass developed at the apex of the vagina. Pathological examination of the uterus showed no choriocarcinoma. Pleuritic pain and hemoptysis soon appeared, and the patient was admitted to NIH on April 1, 1955. The HCG titer was 28,000 units, and a chest x-ray showed one density in each lung, consistent with metastases. Chemotherapy was not available at this time, and she was discharged on April 12, 1955. The HCG titer remained elevated, and repeated chest x-ray examinations showed progression of the pulmonary lesions, new nodules appearing. In July, 1955, headache became a prominent symptom, and in mid-August convulsions and other neurological signs led to readmission on August 26; she died at NIH on August 28, 1955, 8 months after delivery.

Autopsy (A-55–102) of this untreated patient revealed multiple metastases of choriocarcinoma to the brain, with cerebral infarcts and a massive occipital intracerebral hemorrhage, and to the lungs (FIGURE 158), with pulmonary infarcts (FIGURE 159), as well as intravascular emboli of choriocarcinoma in the kidney and vagina (FIGURE 85). Much of the pulmonary choriocarcinoma was in the form of intravascular emboli; however, true metastases were present. One branch of the coronary artery tree was occluded by embolic trophoblast (FIGURE 220) and a small healing myocardial infarct (FIGURE 221) was present in the adjacent area. The uterus was free of tumor. A metastatic nodule was found in the thyroid gland (FIGURE 251). There was diffuse lobular hyperplasia of the breasts (FIGURE 245). The islets of Langerhans were slightly increased in size and number.

Case 5: E.P. (01–87–02), a 30-year-old gravida 5, para 5, had her last term delivery on March 11, 1957. Delayed postpartum bleeding appeared 4 weeks later, and on April 30, 1957, curettage yielded tissue diagnostic of choriocarcinoma. Hysterectomy with bilateral salpingo-oophorectomy was performed 5 days later; the uterus contained a large mass of choriocarcinoma (FIGURE 59). A chest x-ray showed bilateral nodular densities consistent with metastatic lesions. She was treated with nitrogen mustard and x-irradiation to the chest. In August, 1957, a lesion appeared in the vaginal wall, and hemoptysis developed shortly thereafter. She had lost weight and was anemic. She was admitted to NIH on August 14, 1957. The HCG titer on admission was $>$ 1 million units, and a chest x-ray showed extensive pulmonary lesions. Following an initial course of methotrexate therapy, the titer fell to the 5,000–10,000 unit range, but despite three further courses rose to the 1.5–2.0 million unit range. She died on October 8, 1957, with respiratory insufficiency, 7 months postpartum and 2 months after admission.

Autopsy (A-57–204) revealed choriocarcinoma metastatic to both lungs (FIGURE 172), the liver (FIGURE 185), brain, spleen (FIGURES 227 & 228), vagina (FIGURE 86), bladder (ulcerated FIGURE 93), pelvic soft tissue, right gastrocnemius muscle (FIGURE 270), and right kidney. The liver showed diffuse fatty metamorphosis; the breasts were atrophic. There was no evidence of remission.

Case 6: D.T. (02–71–77), an 18-year-old gravida 1, para 1, was delivered of a stillborn infant at term on May 21, 1959. Postpartum bleeding was continuous for 3 months, when successive curettages in August and September, 1959, yielded tissue diagnostic of choriocarcinoma. At hysterectomy on September 10, 1959, a large choriocarcinoma was found invading the uterus; 1 month later pain developed in the occiput and back of the neck, followed by nausea and vomiting, then diplopia. She was admitted to NIH on October 27, 1959. The HCG titer was > 50,000 units, and a chest x-ray showed bilateral nodules consistent with metastatic lesions. Methotrexate therapy was begun on the second hospital day, but on the morning of the fourth hospital day the patient was found unconscious. Neurological examination revealed evidence of a brainstem hemorrhage. The patient died on the seventh hospital day in shock and anuria, less than 6 months after delivery, essentially untreated.

Autopsy (A-59–220) revealed choriocarcinoma metastatic to the lungs (FIGURE 157), cerebellum, dura mater, dome of the bladder, and a retroperitoneal lymph node. The cause of death was a large cerebellar hemorrhage with encephalomalacia. The breasts showed lobular hyperplasia. Acute ulcers were found in the stomach and rectum. Coagulase-positive *Staphylococcus aureus* was recovered from the blood.

Case 7: B.W. (00–77–23), a 30-year-old gravida 4, para 4, had her last term delivery on November 1, 1957. Delayed postpartum bleeding developed 3 weeks later, and curettage on December 15, 1957, yielded tissue suggestive of the histopathological diagnosis of choriocarcinoma. A hysterectomy 3 days later confirmed the diagnosis (FIGURE 63). On January 3, 1958, vaginal hemorrhage requiring packing and suturing developed from secondary vaginal nodules. A chest x-ray showed bilateral pulmonary nodular lesions. She was admitted to NIH on January 16, 1958. The HCG titer was 100,000 units. She received eight courses of methotrexate therapy and the titer declined to 5,000 units by May 9, 1958. After nitrogen mustard therapy was given, the vaginal nodules healed and the roentgenographically demonstrated pulmonary nodules disappeared. She was discharged on May 23, 1958, but readmitted 1 month later when the HCG titer rose and new nodules appeared in a chest x-ray. An additional course of methotrexate therapy was followed by treatment with 2-deoxyglucose and 6-mercaptopurine. Early in August, 1958, signs of central nervous system involvement appeared and gradually progressed. The hypothalamic stalk was sectioned on October 7, but she expired on October 24, 1958, with progressive neurological symptoms, 1 year after delivery and 10 months after admission, having had a temporary therapeutic remission that could not be maintained.

Autopsy (A-58–253) disclosed a solitary metastasis in the right parietal region of the cerebrum, adherent to the dura. Two small nodules contained only hemorrhagic and necrotic material. Organizing thrombi were found in the paravaginal veins.

Case 8: F.T. (03–05–40), a 25-year-old gravida 2, para 1, aborta 1, had her term delivery on January 2, 1960. Gross vaginal hemorrhage occurred 4 weeks later, and a curettage revealed tissue diagnosed as "retained placenta." She was well until May, 1960, when vaginal spotting and fatigue led to hospitalization for a hysterectomy with bilateral salpingo-oophorectomy. A large choriocarcinoma was found invading the uterus. A chest x-ray taken 1 week later showed bilateral nodular densities. She was admitted to NIH on June 22, 1960. The HCG titer was 2 million units, and a bleeding, cauliflower-like mass was present at the vaginal apex. She was given seven courses of methotrexate therapy and two of vincaleukoblastine, with partial clearing of the pulmonary nodules and a decline in the HCG titer to 80,000 units by October, 1960. New pulmonary lesions appeared, however, and the old ones increased in size; the HCG titer rose to levels higher than those on admission. Hematuria became a problem from tumor infiltration of the bladder and contamination of the urine with viable and necrotic tumor cells. She died on December 12, 1960, 11 months after delivery and 6 months after admission, having had a brief partial remission.

Autopsy (A-60–260) disclosed metastatic choriocarcinoma in the vagina, lungs, bladder, and pelvic soft tissue. The deposits contained only small amounts of viable tumor, but there was much hemorrhage, including massive intrapulmonary hemorrhage. There was severe hypoplasia of the bone marrow (FIGURES 241 & 242), and ulcerating, necrotic lesions were found in the tongue, epiglottis (FIGURE 264), trachea, small bowel, and large bowel (FIGURE 208). Fresh hemorrhages were seen in the adrenal glands and renal pelvis (FIGURES 215 & 216); terminal hemothorax and hemoperitoneum were also present. Terminal bacteremia due to gram-negative bacilli, chiefly *Pseudomonas,* was established by both antemortem and postmortem cultures. A nontoxic nodule was found in the thyroid gland.

Case 9: B.G. (03–00–99), an 18-year-old gravida 1, para 1, had her term delivery on February 20, 1960, and continued bleeding. Curettage on May 4 (10 weeks later) showed "endometritis," and bleeding stopped only to recur more severely on May 26, 1960. A second curettage on June 1, 1960 (14 weeks postpartum) showed choriocarcinoma. She was admitted to NIH on June 5, 1960, with an HCG titer of about 1 million units and extensive bilateral nodular deposits seen in a chest x-ray. The titer fell to the range of 20,000–50,000 units, following four courses of methotrexate therapy, and the chest lesions regressed slightly, but two courses of vincaleukoblastine produced no further effect, nor did subsequent courses of methotrexate. Signs of central nervous system involvement became evident in September and progressed despite x-irradiation to the skull. She died on November 2, 1960, a little more than 8 months after delivery and 5 months after admission, having had only a transient, brief remission. The immediate cause of death was massive intraperitoneal hemorrhage.

Autopsy (A-60–234) revealed a large choriocarcinoma replacing most of the uterus with many satellite intramural nodules (FIGURES 18 & 19). It had perforated the uterine wall, infiltrated the broad ligament, and become attached to the omentum and mesentery, incorporating the terminal ileum and appendix (FIGURE 200), finally giving rise to massive hemoperitoneum. A single metastatic nodule was found on the dome of the bladder (FIGURE 92), and there were multiple metastatic nodules in both lungs (FIGURE 148) and a solitary nodule in the brain. A small metastatic deposit was seen in the submucosa of the jejunum. The ovaries were small and showed only minimal luteinization.

Case 10: M.U. (03–86–07), a 27-year-old gravida 3, para 2, aborta 1, had her last term delivery on July 28, 1960. Heavy vaginal spotting necessitated a curettage 4.5 weeks after delivery, and the curettings showed choriocarcinoma. She was transferred to a teaching hospital, where she received 14 courses of methotrexate between October, 1960, and March, 1961. Despite initial improvement, the HCG titer did not fall below 50,000 units. Pelvic masses necessitated hysterectomy and bilateral salpingo-oophorectomy on April 24, 1961. The uterus contained a large mass of choriocarcinoma infiltrating the myometrium widely, and theca-lutein cysts were present in the ovaries. She received two subsequent courses of methotrexate therapy, and was admitted to NIH on October 11, 1961. The HCG titer was between 2 million and 5 million units, and a chest x-ray showed bilateral pulmonary nodular densities. She received four courses of actinomycin D alone, two courses of actinomycin D with chlorambucil, two and one-half courses of leukocristine, and four courses of "triple therapy" consisting of actinomycin D, chlorambucil, and methotrexate. There was no significantly prolonged period of inability to accept medication nor any severe bone marrow toxicity. She became progressively more dyspneic and died on April 31, 1962, 20.5 months after delivery.

Autopsy (A-62–98) disclosed choriocarcinoma metastatic to the lungs, liver, spleen, kidneys (FIGURE 211), diaphragm, retroperitoneal fat, and brain (left parietal and right occipital cortex). Tumor emboli were present in the veins of the pericardial fat, and there was nontumorous thrombophlebitis of major pelvic veins (FIGURE 226). No significant changes were seen in endocrine target organs, nor was there pathological evidence of drug toxicity.

Case 11: L. McD. (03–67–83), a 33-year-old Negro gravida 6, para 5, delivered a stillborn infant at term in November, 1960. Menses resumed but were irregular and heavy. In February, 1961, she developed cough, fatigue, occasional bouts of chills, and fever with night sweats. By April she noted increasing weakness and dyspnea on exertion, and then gastrointestinal bleeding. Gastrointestinal hemorrhage became uncontrolled, and laparotomy was performed on April 27, 1961. A small lesion was removed from the terminal ileum; histopathological examination revealed it to be metastatic choriocarcinoma. A chest x-ray disclosed a large mass in the right lung, and the HCG titer 1 week after intestinal resection was 700,000 units. She was treated with three courses of methotrexate and x-irradiation to the chest, but hemoptysis and gastrointestinal hemorrhage recurred, and new lesions appeared in chest films. A second laparotomy was performed to excise ulcerated metastatic deposits in the small intestine, and she was admitted to NIH on July 14, 1961; the HCG titer was $>$ 5 million units, and chest x-rays confirmed previous observations. She was treated with actinomycin D and then methotrexate, but hemoptysis and gastrointestinal bleeding persisted, and dyspnea and tachypnea became prominent symptoms. Laboratory tests indicated increased thyroid function. She died on August 7, 1961, in respiratory failure, 10 months after delivery.

Autopsy (A-61–187) disclosed metastatic choriocarcinoma in the lungs, heart (FIGURE 219), liver, pancreas, skin, stomach, jejunum, ileum, and kidneys. The uterus contained a nodule of choriocarcinoma within the myometrium. There was no decidual reaction in the endometrium. The ovaries showed no follicle stimulation, but there was a regressing corpus luteum and a few tiny plaques of ectopic decidua beneath the nearby surface mesothelium (FIGURE 103). Minimal lactation changes were seen in the mammary glands. The thyroid gland was normal. A slight degree of Arias-Stella effect was seen in some endometrial glands.

Case 12: A.H. (04–14–30), a 40-year-old gravida 4, para 4, was delivered at term of a female infant in August, 1961. The puerperium was uneventful. A single episode of vaginal bleeding occurred in December, 1961. In January-February, 1962, the patient felt subjective evidence of pregnancy and noted a mass in the right lower quadrant of the abdomen; she had severe "morning sickness." On March 8, 1962, she developed severe left upper quadrant abdominal pain followed by right upper quadrant pain and was hospitalized. Signs of intraperitoneal hemorrhage necessitated laparotomy, which revealed that a huge right ovarian mass had ruptured, spilling blood and tumor freely into the peritoneal cavity and implanting on the sigmoid. Total abdominal hysterectomy, bilateral salpingo-oophorectomy, and segmental resection of sigmoid with removal of all visible tumor implants were performed. A diagnosis of choriocarcinoma was made (FIGURES 80, 81), but the primary site was not determinable. A postoperative HCG level was 400 units. She was admitted to NIH on March 26, 1962; the HCG titer was between 50,000 and 500,000 units, and the chest x-ray on admission was negative. She received three courses of actinomycin D, four courses of methotrexate, and two courses of "triple therapy," but the hormone titer did not decline below the range of 2,000–5,000 units at any time, remaining chiefly between 50,000 and 200,000 units. Abnormal values were obtained on tests for liver function, and a needle biopsy of the liver in May showed fatty metamorphosis. A second laparotomy was performed on October 1, 1962, and choriocarcinoma was found in the parietal peritoneum, but none elsewhere in the abdominal cavity. However, the chest film, which had been negative to this time, showed a nodule in the left midlung field, and the HCG titer rose from the range of 50,000–200,000 units to 2–4 million units, despite three additional courses of "triple therapy" and two courses of vincaleukoblastine during the 3 months following surgery. The chest nodule progressively increased in size to 4 cm in diameter. Her course was progressively downhill, complicated by a *Klebsiella* infection treated with antibiotics, and she died on February 23, 1963, 18 months after delivery.

Autopsy (A-63–53) showed choriocarcinoma metastatic to the lungs, liver, and diaphragm. The deposits in the lung were multiple; many small nodules were present in both lungs. The metastasis in the liver was a large mass 9 cm in diameter, chiefly necrotic. Organized thrombi in pelvic veins were attributed to the two previous operations. [*Note:* No primary site was assigned to this choriocarcinoma. The initial diagnosis was made on tissue from the parametrium at the time of hysterectomy.]

Case 13: N.B. (04–71–49), a 32-year-old gravida 7, para 5, had her last term delivery in 1961, and was in good health with normal menses until July, 1962, when brownish vaginal discharge appeared. She had a normal period on August 7, 1962, following which a 20-day course of norethindrone was given. In September, she experienced severe pain and numbness in the left gluteal area, and then difficulty in urination; the uterus was enlarged. In October, exploration of the pelvis and retroperitoneum showed a hematoma of the left piriformis muscle, but no histological diagnosis was reached. Following surgery, she developed a retroperitoneal hematoma. In November, myelography revealed a filling defect at the level of the first sacral vertebra. She began to pass tarry stools; a chest x-ray at that time showed bilateral nodular densities, and a quantitative Aschheim-Zondek test was reported as "high-normal." On November 13, 1962, severe flank pain and hematuria developed, and a left nephrectomy was performed 6 days later. The kidney was markedly enlarged and two-thirds replaced by tumor that proved to be choriocarcinoma on pathological examination; the primary site was not determined. Theca-lutein cysts were resected from the ovaries. She was admitted to NIH on December 12, 1962; the chest x-ray showed bilateral nodular deposits, and the HCG titer was borderline at 20 million units. She received five courses of actinomycin D, five courses of methotrexate, and a short course of "triple therapy." By the end of April, 1963, the hormone titer was 2,000 units, and there was marked regression of the chest lesions, but she developed signs of toxicity, sepsis, and pneumonia. She became stuporous and was placed in a respirator, finally dying on May 14, 1963, 6 months after the diagnosis of choriocarcinoma was established by left nephrectomy.

Autopsy (A-63–104) showed no evidence of residual choriocarcinoma. The immediate cause of death was acute, hemorrhagic necrotizing bronchopneumonia with nicroabscesses. *Staphylococcus aureus* was cultured from the lungs; the pulmonary nodules were organized and replaced by fibrous tissue, and similar nodules were seen in the right kidney and spleen. Unilateral demyelinization was found in the posterior funiculus of the lumbosacral segment of the spinal cord. Necrotizing ulcers with hemorrhage were found in the epiglottis, trachea, esophagus (FIGURE 205), and small and large intestines. Focal acute myocarditis was present. The liver showed fatty metamorphosis and cholestasis.

Case 14: R.M. (04–45–65), a 32-year-old gravida 5, para 5, delivered a female infant at term on February 2, 1962. Profuse vaginal bleeding developed on March 9, but curettage was unrevealing. Brisk vaginal bleeding recurred on April 3, and was partly controlled by ergotrate, but a second curettage was likewise not diagnostic. Two pregnancy tests were positive on undiluted specimens but negative in all dilutions. She was asymptomatic until June, 1962, when vaginal spotting occurred. An apparently normal period was induced by parenteral neostigmine; 5 days later, norethisterone was given for 20 days. When medication was withdrawn, brisk flow with clots took place, norethisterone administered in increased dosage failed to stop spotting and intermittent bleeding. On July 29, she developed urinary symptoms, and on August 3, examination revealed the uterus to be the size of a 3-month gestation, and a mass was felt bulging into the anterior vaginal wall. A rabbit test was positive at a 1:200 dilution, and a chest x-ray showed secondary deposits in both lower lobes. She was admitted to NIH on August 11, 1962, with a clinical diagnosis of choriocarcinoma. On admission, there was a large, friable vaginal mass and a firm fixed mass in the pelvis. The HCG titer was between 200,000 and 500,000 units, and a chest x-ray confirmed previous findings. An excretory urogram revealed partial ureteral obstruction bilaterally. Significant bleeding developed from the vaginal lesion, and suturing was necessary to control the hemorrhage. She received six courses of methotrexate, with disappearance of the pulmonary lesions, but the hormone titer remained fixed at the range of 5,000–20,000 units. Infection with *Clostridium perfringens* complicated her course in December and January. After intensive antibiotic treatment, hysterectomy was performed on February 27, 1963. The uterus contained a large necrotic mass in which viable foci of neoplastic trophoblast were identified. The necrotic areas contained gram-negative and gram-positive bacteria. The ovaries were not removed. Following hysterectomy, the hormone titer declined to the range of 200–500 units, but by July it had risen again to the 5,000-unit level. Methotrexate therapy had been resumed after surgery, and in May, 1963, "triple therapy" (actinomycin D, chlorambucil, and methotrexate) was begun. In June, an episode of staphylococcal bacteremia occurred. Other complications during the preceding months had been serum hepatitis, prolonged leukopenia, intermittent intestinal obstruction, and a pelvic abscess. She was discharged in partial remission on July 11, 1963, 11 months after first entry.

Between August, 1963, and February, 1964, she had eight further brief admissions to NIH, all with persistently elevated HCG titers and evidence of persistent trophoblastic disease. Despite further chemotherapy, nodules were detected in the chest x-ray in November, 1963, and these gradually increased in size until the time of her final admission in February, 1964. Shortly before entry, she developed abdominal pain. On admission her hematocrit was low, and there was evidence of introabdominal hemorrhage. Despite adequate blood transfusions and chemotherapy with vincaleukoblastine, she died on March 4, 1964, 25 months after term delivery and 19 months after the diagnosis of choriocarcinoma was established.

Autopsy (A-64–39) showed choriocarcinoma metastatic to lungs, brain, liver, and kidney. An hepatic metastasis had ruptured and produced a hemoperitoneum of 2,600 cc. The ovaries were small but showed a subcoelomic ectopic decidual reaction.

Case 15: P.F. (05–57–94), a 34-year-old gravida 3, para 3, delivered a normal infant at term in June, 1962. Menses resumed until December, 1963, when an abnormal bleeding pattern developed. Examination revealed the uterus to be of normal size, and no pelvic abnormalities were found; she was treated with synthetic progestagens until mid-January, 1964. A dry hacking cough developed at this time, and a chest x-ray showed an infiltrate in the left upper lobe, diagnosed as lobar pneumonia and treated unsuccessfully with antibiotics. Vaginal bleeding recurred on February 4, and she was admitted to a university hospital on February 8. The admission chest x-ray showed bilateral nodular densities and left pleural effusion. Bronchoscopy was negative on two occasions, and a scalene lymph node biopsy was also negative. On February 29, an immunological test for pregnancy was positive at 1:1 dilution. On March 2, curettage was performed, and a lung biopsy by thoracotomy; the curettings were not diagnostic, but the lung biopsy showed metastatic choriocarcinoma. She received four courses of methotrexate in March and April, but the immunological tests for pregnancy remained positive at 1:16 dilutions, and there was no roentgenographic evidence of regression of the pulmonary metastases. A grand mal seizure occurred on April 26, and she was admitted to NIH on April 27, 1963. She received four courses of actinomycin D in May without reduction of the HCG titer from admission levels of 200,000–500,000 units, and her respiratory symptoms increased to the point of dyspnea. A course of "triple therapy" was given in June, but respiratory failure progressed and was complicated by evidence of central nervous system involvement. She died on July 1, 1963, 12 months after delivery and 4 months after choriocarcinoma was diagnosed.

Autopsy (A-64–116) disclosed metastatic choriocarcinoma in the lungs, brain, and ascending aorta (FIGURE 223). There was no tumor in the uterus, and the endometrium showed a peculiar reaction similar to that seen with exogenous estrogen-progestagen preparations (FIGURES 76–78). The ovaries showed no cysts, many corpora albicantia, and small plaques of ectopic decidua at the cortical surface (FIGURES 105 & 115); a collar of hilus cells was seen around a small nerve bundle in one ovary (FIGURE 118). Acute ulcerations were present in the small intestine, and there were submucosal hemorrhages in the large bowel and renal pelves. Necrotizing lesions were seen in the trachea. The bone marrow was moderately hypoplastic and showed slight myelofibrosis.

Case 16: F.S. (05–59–64), a 26-year-old Negro gravida 4, para 4, was delivered at term in September, 1962. The puerperium was complicated by postpartum endometritis, which was treated with antibiotics. Menses resumed in October, but were quite prolonged, and intermittent vaginal bleeding continued for a year until late in October, 1963, when she was readmitted because of heavy bleeding. The uterus was enlarged and soft, and the ovaries were enlarged and cystic. Urinary gonadotropins ranged between 45,000 and 90,000 units. After transfusions, a hysterectomy with bilateral salpingo-oophorectomy was performed on November 7, 1963. The uterus contained a large mass of choriocarcinoma penetrating to the serosa, and there was a decidual reaction in the endometrium. Between November, 1963, and April, 1964, she received four courses of methotrexate with only transient reduction in hormone titer to levels of about 10,000 units. Vaginal nodules appeared at the end of April, and cystoscopy revealed lesions in the bladder mucosa; urinary HCG titers rose sharply to 350,000 units. A fifth course of methotrexate was given, and the patient was admitted to NIH on May 8, 1964. Chest x-rays at this time showed multiple bilateral nodular densities. She was treated with five courses of actinomycin D; the pulmonary nodules decreased in size, as did the vaginal implants, and the hormone titer fell to normal levels after 2 months. However, on July 27, as discharge was being considered, she had a grand mal seizure, and a few days later became aphasic, stuporous, and then comatose; hemiparesis and hemianesthesia developed. She died on August 3, 1964, 23 months after delivery and 10 months after choriocarcinoma was diagnosed.

Autopsy (A-64–138) revealed a large solitary metastatic deposit of choriocarcinoma in the left frontal lobe of the brain associated with massive recent hemorrhage. No viable trophoblast was found in the lungs (FIGURE 168) or vagina (FIGURE 91). The trophoblast in both locations had been destroyed.

Case 17: M.W. (04–40–39), a 31-year-old gravida 4, para 4, had a normal term delivery on October 24, 1961. She was rehospitalized 2.5 weeks postpartum because of uterine bleeding and treated by multiple transfusions. There were three admissions between November 11 and December 14, 1961. Laparotomy was performed because of melena, on December 5, 1961; the ileum was found to contain a tumor mass, requiring a segmental resection; pathological diagnosis of the mass was choriocarcinoma. The ovaries were noted to be cystic at laparotomy. A pregnancy test was negative, but a chest x-ray showed a single nodule in the upper lobe of the left lung. She was admitted to the Massachusetts General Hospital on January 8, 1962, where the HCG titer was found to be 4,000 units. She received four courses of methotrexate and three courses of actinomycin D. By July, the findings on chest x-ray were unchanged, but the HCG titer had risen to 50,000 units; she was admitted to NIH on July 18, 1962. She received two further courses of methetrexate, and then five courses of "triple therapy" (methotrexate, chlorambucil, and actinomycin D) with a decline in the hormone titer to 2,000 units. She was discharged on November 15, 1962, scheduled to return for a hysterectomy on November 25. On readmission, the hormone titer was between 200,000 and 500,000 units, and the solitary nodule in the left lung was unchanged. Hysterectomy was deferred on the day following admission because fever had developed. Acute abdominal pain developed, especially marked over the liver and referred to the right shoulder. Blood was aspirated from the right upper quadrant, and the hemoglobin fell to about 8.0 g/100 ml. Despite multiple blood transfusions, intraperitoneal bleeding persisted, and the patient died on December 8, 1962, 14 months after term delivery and 12 months after choriocarcinoma was diagnosed.

Autopsy (A-62–291) revealed choriocarcinoma metastatic to the left lung and liver. The pulmonary metastasis was solitary, largely organized, slightly calcified, and contained minimal viable tumor (FIGURES 170 & 171). The liver contained several small tumor nodules, and there was a subcapsular hematoma containing 800 cc of blood. Hemoperitoneum of 5,000 cc was present. The uterus contained no tumor or decidual reaction, and the ovaries were small.

Case 18: M.C. (04–15–13), a 38-year-old gravida 11, para 7, had a term delivery in October, 1960, at which time tubal ligation was performed. Menses resumed normally until July, 1961, when she developed profuse vaginal bleeding. Following a curettage, which yielded no pathologic diagnosis, she was treated with "hormone injections," which did not control bleeding. She did not continue under medical supervision. In November, 1961, she developed shoulder pain and was treated by a chiropractor. In December, she was hospitalized because of right hemiparesis. The uterus was enlarged; there was an ulcerated lesion in the vagina, a nodule near Skene's gland, and an exophytic lesion on the cervix. A chest x-ray showed multiple diffuse pulmonary nodules and a left pleural effusion. A frog test was positive at 500,000 mouse unit equivalents. Biopsies of the cervical and vaginal lesions were reported as choriocarcinoma. She received six courses of methotrexate. The HCG titer declined to 6,500 units, the hemiparesis cleared completely, the cervical and vaginal lesions healed, and the uterus returned to normal size. The patient gained weight, and her general condition improved. In February, 1962, she was sent home to recuperate before further therapy was planned. After 1 week at home the nodule in Skene's gland had more than doubled in diameter; a biopsy revealed choriocarcinoma. She was admitted to NIH on March 29, 1962. A chest x-ray showed residual nodular densities in both lung fields, and the HCG titer was $>$ 500,000 units. She was considered resistant to methotrexate, and received six courses of actinomycin D, followed by four courses of "triple therapy" (actinomycin D, chlorambucil, and methotrexate). Transient reduction in hormone titers was intermittently achieved, but signs of central nervous system involvement developed in August, and she died on September 6, 1962, 23 months after term delivery and 10 months after the diagnosis of choriocarcinoma was made.

Autopsy (A-62–208) revealed choriocarcinoma metastatic to the lungs, pleura, liver, and serosa of the ileum. A single small nodule of choriocarcinoma was found in the left parovarian region, but the lesions in the uterus, cervix, and vagina were healed. A single metastatic nodule was located between the meninges and cerebral cortex, and there was considerable cerebral edema. Terminal bronchopneumonia was present.

Following Hydatidiform Mole

Case 19: A.A. (02–98–67), a 35-year-old Negro gravida 5, para 4, passed a hydatidiform mole in October, 1958. Vaginal bleeding developed in January, 1959, necessitating hysterectomy, and choriocarcinoma was diagnosed (FIGURES 67 & 68). Apart from mild abdominal discomfort and occasional nausea, she was well until August, 1959, when vaginal bleeding recurred. A vaginal nodule was biopsied and showed choriocarcinoma. The chest x-ray was clear and remained so. Episodic gastrointestinal bleeding supervened with secondary anemia. Therapy consisted of nitrogen mustard and cobalt irradiation to the pelvis. Despite these and supportive measures, the HCG assays remained positive from September, 1959, to March, 1960, when severe gastrointestinal bleeding was treated with methotrexate, and the patient was referred to NIH on May 19, 1960, some 17 months after the diagnosis of choriocarcinoma had been made. On admission, the HCG titer was $>$ 2 million units, and the chest film was clear. Six courses of methotrexate were given, but signs of central nervous system involvement developed, and massive gastrointestinal bleeding recurred. An intestinal resection for jejunal metastasis was carried out on August 15, but the patient succumbed on August 20, 1960, 22 months after the mole was passed and 3 months after admission.

Autopsy (A-60–179) disclosed a large intracerebral hemorrhage in the right frontoparietal area, but no viable choriocarcinoma was demonstrable in the sections of this lesion. Metastatic choriocarcinoma was present in the liver, spleen, left kidney, lungs, jejunum, and omentum. One of the large metastatic nodules in the liver had ruptured, giving rise to terminal intraperitoneal hemorrhage. Diffuse stromal luteinization of the ovaries was present, and the thyroid gland showed focal follicular hyperplasia (FIGURE 253). Diffuse ulcerating lesions were present in the small intestine (FIGURE 206).

Case 20: D.G. (02–47–93), a 35-year-old gravida 5, para 4, was curetted of a hydatidiform mole in October, 1958. A few days later, a hysterectomy was performed, but only a decidual reaction of the endometrium was found. Pregnancy tests remained positive, and in March, 1959, cough and episodic hemoptysis developed. Chest x-rays in April and May disclosed a solitary mass in the right lower lobe, and by the time of admission to NIH on May 28, 1959, she had lost 12 pounds in weight. After three courses of methotrexate therapy, the HCG titer fell from > 2 million units on admission to the range of 2,000–5,000 units, and the solitary mass in the lung was smaller. Two further courses of methotrexate failed to decrease the hormone titer, and the chest lesion remained stable in size and contour. Hemoptysis recurred in August, and the HCG titer rose to 50,000 units. Following two courses of vincaleukoblastine, a right lower lobectomy on October 30 disclosed a large mass of metastatic choriocarcinoma in the lobe (FIGURES 152–156). Neurological signs developed in mid-December, and the HCG titer persisted at preoperative levels despite a transient fall. Over the next 9 months, the patient's condition slowly deteriorated—despite several courses of dichloromethotrexate, podophyllotoxin, and x-irradiation to the chest—as new secondary nodules appeared in chest films. Signs of central nervous system involvement persisted, and liver damage was evidenced by icterus and abnormal liver function tests. She died on September 9, 1960, 23 months after the mole was removed and 15 months after admission.

Autopsy (A-60–199) revealed metastatic choriocarcinoma in both lungs, with extension to the thoracic wall at the lobectomy site, a solitary metastasis to the right frontal area of the cerebral hemisphere, a large metastasis in the liver, and smaller metastases in the thyroid gland and in one vertebral body (FIGURE 235). The ovaries showed an ectopic subcoelomic pseudodecidual reaction and stromal luteinization (FIGURES 98 & 109). Stromal hyperplasia of the breasts was also present (FIGURE 246). The principal cause of death was pulmonary fibrosis secondary to irradiation to the chest.

Case 21: A.H. (00–92–31), a 48-year-old gravida 5, para 4, had her last normal pregnancy in 1945, then menstruated regularly until December, 1957, when persistent vaginal bleeding developed. Curettage in January, 1958, showed a hydatidiform mole, and a hysterectomy with bilateral salpingo-oophorectomy was performed shortly thereafter because of a positive Friedman test and the patient's age. In March she developed dizziness, and in April she complained of right upper quadrant pain, which was followed by fever and anemia. At the beginning of May, she became disoriented and then jaundiced. She was admitted to NIH on May 7, 1958, having received 15 mg of methotrexate orally. A few hours after admission, she became comatose and oliguric, dying 3 days later on May 10, 1958, 5 months after the hydatidiform mole had been removed. She was essentially an untreated case.

Autopsy (A-58–105) revealed metastatic choriocarcinoma to the liver (FIGURE 182), spleen, and diaphragm, as well as embolic choriocarcinoma in pulmonary (FIGURE 162) and renal vessels. A section through the right ventricle showed embolic trophoblast between the trabecular carnae (FIGURE 222). The immediate cause of death was massive intraperitoneal hemorrhage from rupture of a liver metastasis (FIGURE 181). The liver also showed fatty metamorphosis (FIGURE 187). Ulcerative lesions were present on the tongue and esophagus, and the bone marrow was hypoplastic. A noninfiltrating duct-cell carcinoma was found in the left breast, and a follicular adenoma in the thyroid gland. (Histopathological material from the curettage and hysterectomy salpingo-oophorectomy could not be procured).

Case 22: V.H. (02–04–57), a 31-year-old gravida 4, para 2, aborta 1, had a hydatidiform mole (FIGURE 8) evacuated by hysterotomy in November, 1956. Recurrent bleeding led to a curettage in February, 1957, which showed persistent molar villi. Hysterectomy and a right salpingo-oophorectomy in March showed choriocarcinoma invading the uterine wall. Intraperitoneal radioactive gold was given as well as pelvic irradiation. Urinary HCG bioassays were negative until September; a chest x-ray taken at this time showed a solitary nodule in the right upper lobe which was excised and shown to be choriocarcinoma (FIGURE 167). The HCG tests remained negative until July, 1958, when a new nodule appeared in a chest x-ray; she was admitted to NIH on July 8, 1958. The HCG titer was between 300,000 and 1 million units, and the admission chest x-ray confirmed the presence of the pulmonary nodule plus another questionable nodule. Following three courses of methotrexate, the hormone titer fell to 500–1,000 units and the chest x-ray cleared, but anemia and leukopenia persisted. After a fourth course of methotrexate, the hormone titer fell to 200–500 units, and the hemogram was normal. She was discharged on December 21, 1958, but readmitted on February 18, 1959, because of pleuritic pain and dyspnea; a chest x-ray had shown recurrent pulmonary nodules. The HCG titer on readmission was 2,000–5,000 units. Following a fifth course of methotrexate, she developed pancytopenia and acute peritonitis, dying on March 5, 1959, 28 months after the mole was removed and 8 months after her first admission, having had a transient remision.

Autopsy (A-59–52) revealed acute diffuse peritonitis secondary to a perforation of the small intestine, the complication of adhesions following the treatment with radioactive gold. The bone marrow was markedly depleted of hematopoietic elements (FIGURE 239). One small deposit of choriocarcinoma was present in the right lung; it was largely necrotic, and there was extensive intrapulmonary hemorrhage. The breasts showed lobular hyperplasia and perilobular fibrosis. The islets of Langerhans were increased in size and number. There was focal necrosis of scattered glomeruli in both kidneys (FIGURE 217), and microabscesses were found in the psoas muscle (FIGURE 271), secondary to septicemia.

Case 23: B.K. (00–81–79), a 22-year-old gravida 1, had a hydatidiform mole evacuated and bilateral adnexal masses partially resected in February, 1957. The uterus involuted normally, but Aschheim-Zondak tests remained positive to July. Curettages in May, June, and July, 1957, yielded only secretory endometrium and decidua. In July, quantitative Aschheim-Zondak tests and a chest x-ray were negative. In October, there was an episode of vaginal bleeding; the uterus was enlarged and continued to increase. Curettage in November showed choriocarcinoma, and a "coin lesion" was seen on x-ray in the left upper lobe. Vaginal bleeding necessitated multiple transfusions, and the patient was finally admitted to NIH on February 11, 1958. The HCG titer was 4 million units, and the presence of a radiologically solitary chest mass was confirmed. Six courses of methotrexate were given with no appreciable effect. Hyperthyroidism developed, and nitrogen mustard was given. Signs of central nervous system involvement developed, and the patient died on May 30, 1958, 15 months after the mole was removed and almost 4 months after admission, never having had a remission of the disease.

Autopsy (A-58–126) revealed choriocarcinoma primary in the uterus (FIGURE 21), with metastases in the lungs, brain (FIGURE 173), liver, kidneys, and jejunum (FIGURE 198). The thyroid gland showed involution of preceding hyperplasia, and ectopic decidua was found in the ovaries.

Case 24: P.M. (00–90–16), a 23-year-old gravida 1, passed a hydatidiform mole in June, 1956, and was curetted. Vaginal spotting became progressively more severe, and a hysterectomy with bilateral salpingo-oophorectomy was performed in September. A diagnosis of choriocarcinoma of the uterus and multiple theca-lutein cysts of the ovaries was established. Weakness and paresthesias developed in one leg in March, 1957; urinary and bowel symptoms developed in November. Reexploration of the pelvis in January, 1958, disclosed no residual tumor, but neurological symptoms persisted, and myelography revealed a block. Laminectomy was done on March 31, 1958, and tumor tissue was removed; this was followed by local x-irradiation. She was admitted to NIH on April 21, 1958. The HCG titer was between 500,000 and 1 million units, and a chest x-ray showed bilateral scattered mottled densities. After three courses of methotrexate, the hormone titer fell to the range of 4,000–8,000 units, but it rose after a fourth course. Subsequent chemotherapy included 2-deoxyglucose and additional methotrexate, and finally methylcholanthrene endosuccinate. During this period, however, chest lesions increased in number and size, and evidence of central nervous system involvement developed. She died on November 12, 1958, 18 months after the mole was passed and more than 8 months after admission.

Autopsy (A-58–260) revealed metastatic choriocarcinoma in the lungs, tracheobronchial lymph nodes, liver, brain, and epidural space and soft tissue around the lumbar spine, plus an embolus of choriocarcinoma in the right femoral vein and clumps of syncytiotrophoblast in splendic sinusoids. The islets of Langerhans were increased in number and size. The myocardium exhibited focal myocytolysis.

Case 25: B.P. (00–84–21), a 25-year-old gravida 1, was curetted of a hydatidiform mole (FIGURE 6) in July, 1956. Menses resumed normally through November, 1957, when irregular vaginal bleeding appeared. In January, 1958, a frog test was positive, and curettage yielded "trophoblast suspicious for choriocarcinoma," but no villi (FIGURES 51 & 52). Hysterectomy and bilateral salpingo-oophorectomy on February 7, 1958, showed choriocarcinoma of the uterus (FIGURES 69 & 70) and theca-lutein cysts of the ovaries. Dysplastic changes were seen in the squamous epithelium of the exocervix (FIGURE 84). A chest x-ray showed nodular lesions that increased in size, and a nodule appeared in the vagina later that month. She was admitted to NIH on March 3, 1958. The HCG titer was 4 million units, and chest films showed extensive bilateral secondary deposits. After ten courses of methotrexate, the hormone titer fell to 10,000 units, and the pulmonary lesions stabilized but did not clear completely. She was discharged on August 2, 1958, to the care of her referring physicians, who gave two more courses of methotrexate; the vaginal nodule reappeared in November, and signs of central nervous system involvement appeared. These progressed rapidly, and she died on November 27, 1958, 28 months after the mole was removed and 9 months after first admission, having had only a partial remission.

Autopsy (A-58–278) revealed choriocarcinoma metastatic to the lungs, spleen (FIGURE 229), brain, vagina, and a pelvic lymph node near the bladder. The pulmonary metastases were very necrotic and hemorrhagic; the cerebral metastases were multiple in the left hemisphere. The islets of Langerhans were increased in number and size. There was necrosis of the pituitary gland (FIGURES 259 & 260) and focal necrosis in the adrenal cortex. Toxic changes were seen in the ileal mucosa.

Case 26: B.R. (02–04–77), a 35-year-old gravida 2, para 1, had a term delivery on June 6, 1955, and was curetted of a hydatidiform mole on November 10, 1955. Vaginal bleeding in January, 1956, necessitated curettage, and retained molar tissue was evacuated. A Friedman test was positive in February, but negative in April. Intermittent irregular vaginal spotting and brownish discharge continued to January, 1958, several Friedman tests being negative and two curettages failing to yield trophoblastic tissue. Late in January, 1958, she developed pain in the anterior chest and epigastrium. A chest x-ray showed nodular densities in both lungs, and nitrogen mustard was given in February. In March, a Friedman test was positive; a hysterectomy with bilateral salpingo-oophorectomy was performed on March 6, 1958. A diagnosis of choriocarcinoma invading the uterus was established, and the ovaries showed theca-lutein cysts and stromal luteinization, as well as ectopic decidual plaques. She received four courses of methotrexate, then additional nitrogen mustard therapy, and a course of methotrexate at higher dosage. She was admitted to NIH on July 9, 1958. The HCG titer was 4,400,000 units, and the chest x-ray showed diffuse bilateral pulmonary nodules. Three more courses of methotrexate and two courses of 2-deoxyglucose failed to produce remission. Signs of central nervous system involvement developed, and she died on October 13, 1958, 35 months after the mole was removed and 3 months after admission.

Autopsy (A-58–234) showed metastatic choriocarcinoma to the lungs, brain, liver, right adrenal gland (FIGURES 256 & 257), and left kidney (FIGURE 214). The immediate cause of death was intracerebral and subarachnoid hemorrhage from a solitary metastasis in the left parietooccipital lobe. An organizing hemorrhagic infarct was present in the anterior lobe of the pituitary gland.

Case 27: D.S. (01–91–61), a 23-year-old gravida 2, para 1, was curetted of a hydatidiform mole in February, 1956, and was well until August, 1957, when hemoptysis occurred. After another episode of hemoptysis 3 weeks later, a chest x-ray showed two or three isolated pulmonary nodules. A Friedman test was positive, similar tests having been previously negative. Frontal headaches, vomiting, blurring of vision, and papilledema developed, and she was admitted to NIH on September 20, 1957. The HCG titer was $>$ 4 million units, and a chest x-ray showed three secondary nodules. After seven courses of methotrexate, the hormone titer fell to the range of 2,500–5,000 units; the chest films and neurological signs improved. She was discharged on pass on December 19, 1957, but readmitted with her HCG titer elevated to 2 million units and a vaguely defined pelvic mass on January 4, 1958. Another course of methotrexate was followed by nitrogen mustard and DON (6-diazo-5-oxo-L-leucine), but neurological signs reappeared early in March. Two courses of intravenous and intrathecal methotrexate were given, but the patient's condition deteriorated and she died on April 20, 1958, 26 months after the mole was removed and 7 months after admission, having had only a transient partial remission.

Autopsy (A-58–83) showed choriocarcinolma metastatic to the lungs, liver, pancreas (FIGURE 188), spleen, and right adrenal gland, and a solitary metastatic nodule in the right cerebral hemisphere (FIGURE 176). Thrombosis was present in the mesenteric venous drainage (FIGURE 224). No choriocarcinoma was found in the uterus, and the endometrium did not show a decidual reaction. Plaques of ectopic decidua and theca-lutein cysts were present on the ovary; hilar cell hyperplasia was deteced (FIGURE 117).

Case 28: E.W. (02–70–80), a 34-year-old gravida 5, para 2, aborta 2, passed a hydatidiform mole in January 1959, and 2 weeks later underwent a hysterectomy with bilateral salpingo-oophorectomy. There was no tumor in the uterus. She remained well and asymptomatic until September, when she developed pain in the right lower chest and abdomen. A chest x-ray showed bilateral nodular densities, and a Friedman test was positive. Severe vomiting supervened, and she was admitted to NIH on October 20, 1959; the HCG titer was over 1 million units. Signs of acute intraperitoneal bleeding had developed while the patient was en route. She developed shock and anuria, dying 4 days after admission, untreated.

Autopsy (A-59–210) showed choriocarcinoma metastatic to the lungs and liver. The massive intraperitoneal hemorrhage came from rupture of one of the liver metastases. There was hyperplasia of the islets of Langerhans (FIGURE 190) and a small, discrete islet-cell adenoma (FIGURE 189). Lobular hyperplasia, secretory vacuoles, and intraluminal secretions were found in the breast tissue (FIGURE 248).

Case 29: M.P. (03–14–75), a 32-year-old gravida 1, had a hydatidiform mole evacuated by hysterotomy in February, 1958, and a cystic right ovary was removed at that time. Menses resumed normally until September, 1959, when menometrorrhagia led to a curettage in October, which revealed normal endometrium. An Aschheim-Zondak test was positive, and a hysterectomy with left salpingo-oophorectomy was performed in November; the endometrium was in the proliferative phase, and the ovary was unremarkable. She remained well until July, 1960, when she developed cough and pain in the right shoulder. Hemoptysis occurred in August, and a chest x-ray showed bilateral pulmonary nodules. She was admitted to NIH on August 23, 1960. The HCG titer was between 2 million and 5 million units. Despite prolonged therapy with methotrexate (nine courses), vincaleukoblastine, leukocristine, DON (6-diazo-5-oxo-L-leucine), and "triple therapy" (consisting of combined methotrexate, chlorambucil and actinomycin D), her titer persisted at high levels, and the chest lesions did not regress. Severe liver damage from either drugs or serum hepatitis occurred and progressed to chronic liver disease, and she finally died on February 11, 1962, 48 months after the mole was removed and almost 18 months after admission, having had no significant remission.

Autopsy (A-62–33) revealed choriocarcinoma metastatic to the lungs, brain (FIGURE 174), liver, anterior mediastinum, and both adrenal glands. Tumor emboli were present in the left renal vein and central vein of the left adrenal gland (FIGURE 255). The liver showed subacute hepatitis with posthepatitic cirrhosis (FIGURE 183). Central focal necrosis was present in the anterior pituitary (FIGURE 261), and the thyroid gland showed focal involution and interstitial fibrosis.

Case 30: C.R. (02–69–34), a 24-year-old gravida 1, passed a hydatidiform mole in August, 1958. Vaginal spotting occurred in October, and a curettage yielded no trophoblastic tissue. Vaginal bleeding recurred in February, 1959, and the HCG titer was 200,000 units. A hysterectomy with bilateral salpingo-oophorectomy was performed; the uterus showed a zone of superficial necrosis but no trophoblastic lesion. The ovary showed a theca-lutein reaction (FIGURES 95–97). She was well until September, when hemoptysis occurred. A chest film showed questionable secondary deposits, and she was admitted to NIH on October 10, 1959. The HCG titer was between 2 million and 4 million units, and the chest x-ray was equivocal. She was treated for 32 months with ten courses of methotrexate alone, two courses of vincaleukoblastine, three courses of actinomycin D plus chlorambucil, five courses of actinomycin D alone, and one course of nitrogen mustard, plus cyclophosphamide, methyl GAG (glyoxal bis(guanylhydrazone), DON (6-diazo-5-oxo-L-leucine), and podophyllotoxin. Despite transient fluctuations, the hormone titer never declined significantly, and multiple pulmonary lesions gradually appeared in the chest x-rays and increased in size. She died on June 9, 1962, without having had a remission, 46 months after passing the mole and 32 months after admission.

Autopsy (A-62–134) revealed choriocarcinoma almost completely replacing the left lung and multiple nodules in the right lung. Multiple metastases were found in the brain, small bowel (FIGURE 197) and mesenteric lymph nodes, spleen, and both kidneys (FIGURE 210). A large tumor thromboembolus partially obstructed the main left pulmonary artery (FIGURE 225). Pronounced lobular hyperplasia was present in breast tissue (FIGURE 247). Bacteremia was present terminally, and *Pseudomonas* was recovered from the postmortem blood cultures.

Case 31: R.G. (02–55–95), a 24-year-old Negro gravida 4, para 3, passed a hydatidiform mole (FIGURE 2) on July 12, 1958. Vaginal bleeding continued, and the Aschheim-Zondak (A-Z) test was positive on September 22. Vaginal bleeding recurred, and a second curettage on October 2 yielded atypical trophoblastic tissue with an Arias-Stella reaction (FIGURE 79). A hysterectomy was performed on October 24, 1958, and a chorioadenoma destruens was found in the left uterine cornu (FIGURES 3 & 4). Molar villi had invaded the uterine wall and were surrounded by sheets of proliferated trophoblast which had further invaded. An A-Z test was positive on November 30, and a chest x-ray was clear. In January, 1959, another A-Z test was positive, and in February 1959, nodular deposits were seen in a chest x-ray for the first time. She received five courses of methotrexate, and the A-Z test reverted to negative by April, but the nodules persisted in the lungs unchanged. Icterus developed in May, and a needle biopsy helped establish the diagnosis of viral hepatitis. She received four more courses of methotrexate, but the pulmonary nodules did not change, and the A-Z test became positive by July. She was admitted to NIH on July 11, 1959. Lenkopenia from the previous courses of methotrexate was present, and the HCG titer was between 100,000 and 1 million units. The hormone titer declined to 20,000–50,000 units by July 22 without medication, but then rose to preadmission levels. Following a course of methotrexate therapy, the pulmonary nodules increased in size; three courses of vincaleukoblastine were given and the chest lesions became stable, but the hormone titer rose to 2 million units. Hemothorax developed in October and persisted despite thoracentesis and more vincaleukoblastine. In January, 1960, an intravenous pyelogram indicated the presence of a large intrapelvic mass. She was discharged unimproved on February 9, 1960, and died at another hospital on March 26, 1960, 20 months after passing the mole and 9 months after admission.

Autopsy† (A-61–53) showed choriocarcinoma metastatic to both lungs, the liver (FIGURE 5), and the spleen. The metastasis in the liver was a large mass, 15 cm in diameter, in the right lobe. Arising from the right parametrium was a large mass (15×10 cm) that almost filled the pelvis and was adherent to the ileum. [*Note:* This case is interpreted as choriocarcinoma developing from a chorioadenoma destruens.]

Case 32: M.R. (00–86–02), a 51-year-old gravida 4, para 2, aborted after a 3-month gestation in 1953, and was told she had had a hydatidiform mole. Following this, she experienced amenorrhea until December, 1957, when continuous vaginal bleeding began. A hysterectomy with bilateral salpingo-oophorectomy was performed in January, 1958, and diagnosed as choriocarcinoma invading the uterus. Dyspnea developed in March, 1958, and two vaginal nodules appeared; she was admitted to NIH on March 16, 1958. The HCG titer was $>$ 100,000 units, and a chest x-ray showed bilateral pulmonary nodules. She received one course of methotrexate, but failed rapidly as dyspnea progressed, and she died 12 days after admission.

Autopsy (A-58–68) showed choriocarcinoma extensively metastatic to both lungs, with considerable necrosis. Metastases were also found in the vagina, bladder, and mediastinal lymph nodes. A small metastasis was present in the brain. Necrotizing lesions were found on the skin and in the mouth. [*Note:* The clinical history of a mole 4 years before the onset of the present illness followed by 4 years of complete amenorrhea is unusual. One cannot be certain whether the choriocarcinoma developed from the trophoblast of the mole or from a new pregnancy that presented as an abortion in December, 1957.]

Case 33: F.J. (01–38–01), a 35-year-old gravida 3, para 2, passed a hydatidiform mole (FIGURES 9 & 10), which was further evacuated by hysterotomy on October 27, 1953. She was well until December, 1954, when she had severe vaginal bleeding and passed a decidual cast. At this time, the chest x-ray was clear and the uterus was small. In June, 1956, she complained of vaginal bleeding over the previous 5 weeks, and a chest film showed multiple large nodules in both lung fields; a Friedman test was positive. She was admitted to NIH on July 23, 1956; the HCG titer was 50,000 units. Curettage on August 7 yielded proliferative endometrium, and a hysterectomy with bilateral salpingo-oophorectomy on August 14 also failed to disclose uterine choriocarcinoma. Postoperatively, she developed intermittent intestinal obstruction, and a segment of jejunum was resected on September 4; the specimen showed evi-

†Autopsy was performed at the United States Naval Hospital, Charleston, S.C. (A-19–60).

dence of intussusception and metastatic choriocarcinoma. Signs of central nervous system involvement developed following the operation, and craniotomy on September 16 revealed choriocarcinoma metastatic to the cerebrum. She received methotrexate (50 mg daily) on September 16, 17, and 18, but died on September 19, 1956, 35 months after the hydatidiform mole was passed, and is included among the "untreated" cases.

Autopsy (A-56–158) revealed metastatic choriocarcinoma in both lungs, the brain, and small intestine (FIGURE 201), with one metastasis to a mesenteric lymph node (FIGURE 233). There was mild hyperplasia of the breast lobules, and the islets of Langerhans (FIGURE 191) were increased in number and size. Examination of the ovaries removed previously showed ectopic decidua, hilar cell hyperplasia, stromal hyperplasia, and a minimal theca-lutein reaction.

Case 34: R.C. (03–50–89), a 23-year-old gravida 3, para 0, had spontaneous abortions in 1956, 1957, and the last in May, 1958, which was a hydatidiform mole. Menses resumed normally until her admission to NIH in April, 1961. However, in December, 1960, she had had two episodes of hemoptysis. Chest x-rays revealed a lesion in the lower lobe of the right lung which was interpreted as a granuloma and treated with antibiotics. Nonproductive cough and occasional blood-streaked sputum persisted. Antibiotic therapy failed to produce regression of the chest lesion; in fact, satellite nodules appeared. Thoracotomy was performed on March 31, 1961, and a "huge, bluish-red soft mass which occupied the entire apex of the right lower lobe" was removed by lobectomy. Satellite nodules were present in this lobe as well as in wedges removed from the right upper lobe. Histopathological examination proved the tumor to be choriocarcinoma. A frog pregnancy test on serum following surgery was reported as negative. She was admitted to NIH on April 15, 1961. The HCG titer was between 200,000 and 500,000 units, and a chest x-ray showed residual nodules in the right lung as well as nodules in the left lung. She developed a nodule in the lower gingiva which was biopsied and also proved to be metastatic choriocarcinoma (FIGURE 193). She received three courses of methotrexate, four courses of actinomycin D alone, and three courses of actinomycin D with chlorambucil. Her course was complicated by persistent vaginal bleeding, and then anemia after the bleeding was controlled. Chemical evidence of liver damage was present for about a month before death. Shortly before death, she was given a brief course of leucocristine, following which she developed severe leukopenia. She died on September 26, 1961, 6 months after lobectomy.

Autopsy (A-61–225) revealed metastatic choriocarcinoma in the lungs, liver, stomach, ileum, kidneys, spleen, brain (FIGURE 175), and right ovary (FIGURES 119 & 120). Neither ovary showed any follicle stimulation or luteinization. A patchy, weak decidual reaction was present in the endometrium, but no tumor was found in the uterus. Mild lactation changes were present in the mammary glands. The liver showed sever fatty metamorphosis (FIGURE 184) and focal hemorrhages, and the mucosa of the small intestine was atrophic (FIGURE 207). Focal necrosis and siderosis was found in the bone marrow (FIGURE 243). A moderate amount of gastrointestinal hemorrhage was present. The major cause of death was a toxic reaction to chemotherapy.

Case 35: A.K. (05–58–81), a 48-year-old gravida 1, para 0, passed a hydatidiform mole in October, 1962, and was curetted. The Friedman test was positive 2 months later but negative after 3 months. In November, 1963, vaginal bleeding recurred and was controlled by hormone injections. Vaginal bleeding recurred in February, 1964, and a curettage in March showed decidua and trophoblast. Dyspnea, chills, fever, and hemoptysis soon developed, and a chest x-ray showed infiltration in both lower lung fields. The uterus was enlarged to the size of a 3-to-4-month gestation. She was admitted to NIH on April 30, 1964; the HCG titer was between 200,000 and 500,000 units. She received five courses of methotrexate with only slight response, then three courses of actinomycin D alone, then four courses of "triple therapy." She exhibited severe toxic responses to the second and third regimens, and her hormone titer never declined below 5,000 units for more than an occasional single determination. There was no significant clearing of the nodular densities in the chest film. Following a short discharge over Christmas in 1964, she was readmitted on January 23, 1965, with profound weakness and dyspnea. The HCG titer was $>$ 500,000 units, and a chest film showed multiple large nodules and diffuse infiltration bilaterally. She died in respiratory failure on January 25, 1965, 23 months after the hydatidiform mole was passed.

Autopsy (A-65–15) showed choriocarcinoma of the uterus, with multiple metastases in both lungs replacing most of the pulmonary parenchyma. Other metastases were in the liver, kidney, jejunum, and a lumbar vertebra; a small tumor nodule was found in the skin of the shoulder (FIGURES 265–267), and there was a solitary metastasis in the right parietal lobe of the brain. The liver showed postnecrotic cirrhosis with patchy fatty metamorphosis. There was a mild increase in size and number of the islets of Langerhans (FIGURE 192). The ovaries were normal in size and free of cysts or cystic follicles; germ cells were not seen in routine sections. There was diffuse increase of both cortical and medullary ovarian stroma, but no theca-lutein reaction or cysts (FIGURE 99). The bone marrow was the site of old and recent hemorrhage (FIGURE 237).

Following Abortion

Case 36: A.M. (02–76–88), a 36-year-old gravida 3, para 2, had a spontaneous abortion on March 24, 1957, and was curetted. Menses resumed but became irregular in October, 1958. A second curettage on January 27, 1959, showed "retained products of conception." Bleeding continued, and a vaginal hysterectomy on April 13, 1959, was reported as showing "probable cervical pregnancy and mild nonspecific endometritis." In October, 1959, a mass developed in the right neck, and severe gastrointestinal bleeding followed. At laparotomy on November 6, 1959, a loop of jejunum, the spleen, and a portion of the liver were resected. Methotrexate therapy was started intravenously in the recovery room after a frozen section had returned a diagnosis of choriocarcinoma. After two courses of methotrexate, the patient was transferred to NIH on December 6, 1959; icterus had developed and was progressing. The HCG titer was > 2 million units, but a chest x-ray was clear. After two additional courses of methotrexate, the hormone titer declined to 20,000–50,000 units, but jaundice deepened and sepsis appeared. The patient died on January 18, 1960, 34 months after the abortion and 6 weeks after admission.

Autopsy (A-60–16) showed choriocarcinoma metastatic to the lungs, liver, small intestine (FIGURE 199), and kidney. Severe fatty metamorphosis of the liver was also present, as well as acute and chronic pyelonephritis. Postmortem blood culture yielded *Pseudomonas*. The ovary showed an ectopic decidual reaction but no luteinization.

Case 37: D.P. (00–94–03), a 47-year-old gravida 1, had a spontaneous abortion on September 4, 1957, and was curetted. Vaginal bleeding recurred on January 1, 1958. A positive frog test was followed by a second curettage on January 23, which yielded a diagnosis of choriocarcinoma, confirmed by hysterectomy and bilateral salpingo-oophorectomy 4 days later. A right parametrial mass was detected in April, and urinary symptoms developed. A vaginal nodule was biopsied on April 24 and showed choriocarcinoma. Massive hematuria developed, and she was admitted to NIH on May 20, 1958. A right nephrectomy was performed on May 26, and the kidney contained a large metastasis. The HCG titer was 20,000–40,000 units and the chest x-ray was clear. A single course of methotrexate was given from May 27 to May 31, but agranulocytosis developed, followed by sepsis and death on June 8, 1958, 8 months after the abortion and 3 weeks after admission.

Autopsy (A-58–133) revealed a few small secondary deposits of choriocarcinoma in the lungs; they were almost completely necrotic and surrounded by bacterial colonies (FIGURE 169). A thrombus of viable choriocarcinoma lined the left external iliac vein, but no other trophoblastic elements were found. The bone marrow was severely aplastic. The vaginal lesion was diffusely necrotic, possibly a portal of entry for bacteria, but necrotizing, ulcerated lesions were also present in the mouth, tongue, and pharynx. Gram-negative bacilli and gram-positive cocci were recovered from postmortem blood cultures. A microfollicular adenoma was found in the thyroid gland.

Case 38: F.S. (00–14–85), a 27-year-old gravida 3, para 2, was curetted after a spontaneous abortion on October 6, 1953. The degree of trophoblastic hyperplasia was considered atypical. An Aschheim-Zondak test was positive on November 2, and a second curettage yielded tissue consistent with choriocarcinoma. Hysterectomy and bilateral salpingo-oophorectomy on December 13 showed choriocarcinoma invading the uterus (FIGURE 56), and the ovaries showed a stromal luteinization (FIGURES 112, 113) and hilar cell hyperplasia. In January, 1954, low-back pain with sciatic distribution developed and progressed to paralysis. She was admitted to NIH on April 23, 1954; the HCG titer was between 100,000 and 500,000 units. X-Irradiation to the mid-back was given, plus large doses of cortisone. Dyspnea and right-sided congestive heart failure developed, and she died on August 12, 1954, "untreated" and without remission, 10 months after the abortion and 5 months after admission.

Autopsy (A-54–38) revealed choriocarcinoma metastatic to the lungs, with diffuse obstruction of the pulmonary artery tree by tumor emboli (FIGURES 164–166) as well as large parenchymatous nodules. A metastatic deposit was found involving the lumbar vertebrae (FIGURE 236), psoas muscle, and epidural space with infarction of the spinal cord. The adrenal cortices were narrowed and depleted of lipid secondary to cortisone therapy. Cor pulmonale and diffuse passive congestion of viscera were consistent with the terminal clinical picture. The pituitary gland showed patchy necroses in the anterior lobe (FIGURE 258).

Case 39: R.T. (01–92–40), a 36-year-old Negro gravida 5, para 4, had her last menstrual period in October, 1956. Following a missed period in November, she began to have intermittent vaginal bleeding in December which continued to June, 1957, when curettage established a diagnosis of choriocarcinoma; a hysterectomy with bilateral salpingo-oophorectomy a few days later showed choriocarcinoma infiltrating the uterus. A chest film showed bilateral nodular densities. Vaginal spotting continued, and in September a vaginal nodule was excised. She was admitted to NIH on September 25, 1957; the HCG titer was 5 million units, and the chest x-ray showed many large nodular densities. Following several courses of methotrexate in various dosages, the hormone titer fell to the level of 5,000–10,000 units by December. However, signs of central nervous system involvement appeared, and the titer rose to the 75,000–100,000 units range. She was treated with DON (6-diazo-5-oxo-L-leucine) in January, 1958, then 5-fluorouracil in February, plus a final instillation of methotrexate into a ventriculostomy catheter, but died on March 1, 1958, 14 months after the abortion and 5 months after admission.

Autopsy (A-58–40) showed choriocarcinoma metastatic to the lungs, liver, right kidney, spleen, subcutaneous tissue of the chest wall near a rib (FIGURE 234), and brain. The cervix showed atypical squamous metaplasia and "pregnancy" changes in the endocervical glands (FIGURE 83). The ovaries showed ectopic decidua but no theca-lutein reaction. The inferior vena cava contained a nonocclusive thrombus.

Case 40: J.J. (02–40–87), an 18-year-old gravida 1, whose last menstrual period was in July, 1958, had a spontaneous abortion on January 6, 1959. Intermittent vaginal bleeding persisted, and a curettage on March 10, 1959, yielded tissue diagnostic of choriocarcinoma (FIGURE 44). An attack of "asthma" on March 30 led to a chest x-ray that showed bilateral nodular densities. She was admitted to NIH on April 4, 1959; the HCG titer was between 2 million and 4 million units. After six courses of methotrexate the titer fell to 20,000–50,000 units, but the chest x-rays did not show resolution of the nodules. Four courses of vincaleukoblastine, a seventh course of methotrexate, and two courses of cyclophosphamide failed to induce response, and the hormone titer rose to 4 million units by mid-August. Hysterectomy and bilateral salpingo-oophorectomy on September 28 revealed choriocarcinoma in the uterus. Anemia and signs of central nervous system involvement developed, and she died on November 11, 1959, 11 months after abortion and 7 months after admission, essentially unremitted.

Autopsy (A-59–227) showed choriocarcinoma metastatic to the lungs (FIGURES 146 & 147), liver, brain, and adrenal (FIGURE 254) and thyroid glands. The immediate cause of death was acute mediastinitis secondary to rupture of the esophagus (FIGURE 195) from vomiting (Boerhaave's syndrome). The hysterectomy specimen (S-59–1936) showed choriocarcinoma invading the uterus (FIGURES 22–24). The ovaries showed a few cystic follicles lined up in a row beneath the cortex, but there was no luteinization, ectopic, decidua, or hilar cell hyperplasia. The curettings from which choriocarcinoma was diagnosed (S-59–889) showed an Arias-Stella effect.

Case 41: G.D. (04–35–19), a 41-year-old gravida 5, para 3, aborted spontaneously after about 20 weeks of gestation on August 12, 1961. Pathological examination of the tissue passed showed no evidence of hydatidiform mole or choriocarcinoma. Uterine bleeding persisted, and a curettage about 1 month after the abortion yielded tissue diagnosed as an organizing placental remnant. Uterine bleeding recurred in November, 1961, 3 months after the abortion; the uterus was felt to be still somewhat enlarged, and another curettage yielded tissue diagnostic of choriocarcinoma; a frog test was positive. Hysterectomy and bilateral salpingo-oophorectomy performed later that month revealed two nodules of choriocarcinoma in the uterus; the ovaries were described as atrophic (FIGURE 108). A chest x-ray in January, 1962, was negative. In March, she developed chest pain, cough, and dyspnea, and a chest film showed bilateral nodular densities in both lung fields, consistent with metastatic choriocarcinoma. She was treated with several courses of methotrexate in varying dosage schedules [precise data regarding dosage and effect on pregnancy tests is lacking]. She was admitted to NIH on July 1, 1962, at which time the HCG titer was between 2 million and 5 million units. A chest x-ray showed extensive nodular pulmonary deposits. A large, fixed mass was present in the left pelvis. Signs and symptoms of urinary tract infection were present, and the presence of left ureteral obstruction and left pyonephrosis due to *Proteus vulgaris* was established. She was treated with antibiotics and six courses of actinomycin-D. Her course was complicated by sepsis secondary to her urinary tract infection and hepatotoxicity. In October, 1962, she was treated with methotrexate (20 mg intramusculary daily) for 6 days, but she developed severe bone marrow depression. She finally died on October 26, 1962, with icterus, coma, and sepsis, 14 months after abortion and 11 months after choriocarcinoma was diagnosed.

Autopsy (A-62–255) revealed choriocarcinoma metastatic to the pelvis, lungs, and spinal cord (FIGURE 179). Postmortem cultures of blood and liver yielded *Pseudomonas* and hemolytic *Staphylococcus aureus*. Moniliasis involving the vagina, urethra, bladder, ureters, kidneys, and large bowel was also present. The kidneys showed acute and chronic pyelonephritis. The liver showed necrosis and centrilobular hemorrhage. Ulcers were present on the epiglottis (FIGURES 262 & 263), esophagus (FIGURE 204), and large and small intestinal mucosa. The bone marrow showed severe depletion of all cellular elements (FIGURE 238).

Case 42: J.K. (04–50–36), a 31-year-old gravida 5, para 2, aborta 1, ectopic 1, became pregnant for the fifth time in November, 1960. Irregular vaginal bleeding from January through April, 1961, led to a curettage in April, and the tissue was diagnosed as "degenerating fetal and placental products" [these sections were not available for review at NIH]. Between April and September, 1961, irregular bleeding continued and three curettages were performed; the curettings were described as abundant and diagnosed grossly as imcomplete abortion; no microscopical studies were performed. She was hospitalized briefly for acute pyelonephritis in early September, then readmitted later that month for severe vaginal bleeding. Curettage yielded large chunks of firm tissue diagnosed on microscopical examination as choriocarcinoma. The HCG assay was reported as 150,000 units; a chest x-ray showed no secondary deposits. Hysterectomy with bilateral salpingo-oophorectomy was performed on September 28, 1961; the specimen showed choriocarcinoma infiltrating the uterus and bilateral ovarian theca-lutein cysts. Following surgery, the HCG titer fell to 5,000 units. A course of oral methotrexate was given. In January, 1962, a questionable nodule appeared on a chest x-ray, and multiple nodules were present by March; the hormone titer had risen to 500,000 units. From March through July, she received irradiation to the chest; in August, two courses of vincaleukoblastine were given, but urinary assays for HCG continued positive in various dilutions. She was finally admitted to NIH on September 3, 1962. The HCG titer was about 50,000 units, and the chest film showed multiple bilateral nodules. She received three courses of actinomycin-D, five courses of "triple therapy," three courses of vincaleukoblastine, and two preterminal courses of methotrexate in high dosage. Her course was complicated by recurrent urinary tract infection, considerable drug toxicity, seizures and hemiparesis, evidence of hepatic damage, and gastrointestinal bleeding. Despite medication, the pulmonary lesions increased in size and number; the HCG titers declined transiently, but rose to even higher levels, attaining a peak of 20 million units preterminally. She finally expired on April 11, 1963, in respiratory failure and with signs of central nervous system involvement, 19 months after choriocarcinoma was diagnosed and 24 months after the curettage for incomplete abortion.

Autopsy (A-63–88) showed choriocarinoma metastatic to the lungs, liver (FIGURE 180), brain (FIGURE 177), spleen, left kidney, stomach, jejunum, ileum, colon, dura mater, and mesenteric and pulmonary hilar lymph nodes. Acute bronchopneumonia with microabscesses was present. Acute fibrinous pericarditis and pleurities were found. There were terminal focal hemorrhages in the stomach, cecum, and right renal calyces. The bone marrow showed panhypoplasia.

Type of Antecedent Gestation not Certain

Case 43: H.K. (00–89–02), a 31-year-old gravida 4, para 3, had a hydatidiform mole in September, 1954, and a term delivery in August, 1956. Menses resumed normally until July, 1957. Despite two curettages, bleeding did not stop, and no histopathological diagnosis could be made. In January, 1958, she developed headache, visual disturbances, and vomiting. Hysterectomy was performed on February 23, 1958, but no tumor was found. Craniotomy on March 24, 1958, revealed choriocarcinoma metastatic to the occipital lobe. She was admitted to NIH on April 9, 1958, deeply jaundiced. The HCG titer was between 500,000 and 1 million units; the chest x-ray showed multiple bilateral. One course of methotrexate was given; sore throat, diarrhea, increasing jaundice, and hemorrhagic phenomena developed, and she died with pancytopenia and bacteremia 9 days after admission.

Autopsy (A-58–62) showed multiple cerebral metastases of choriocarcinoma was well as metastases to the lungs, liver, and jejunum. Tumor emboli were present in the branches of the splenic artery and the right renal artery. The ovaries (FIGURE 100) showed focal ectopic decidua, minimal luteinization, and a "micropolycystic" configuration. Islet-cell hyperplasia was found in the pancreas. The bone marrow was aplastic (FIGURE 240). Necrotizing and hemorrhagic ulcerations were found in the mouth, tongue (FIGURE 202), esophagus (FIGURE 203), and jejunum; pseudomembranous enterocolitis was present in the ileum and large bowel.

Case 44: V.C. (05–89–03), a 33-year-old gravida 1, para 1, with a history of irregular menses and infertility, missed her period in December, 1963. She thought she was pregnant, but in January, 1964, irregular vaginal bleeding developed and continued for 3 months. On April 6, 1964, dilatation and curettage yielded proliferative endometrium. She had an apparently normal menstrual period in May, but from June through September experienced intermittent episodes of irregular bleeding. Profuse vaginal bleeding began on October 2, 1964, and 2 weeks later an egg-shaped mass appeared at the vaginal introitus. She was admitted to the hospital on October 20 with a hemoglobin of 6.9 g/100 ml; curettage again revealed proliferative endometrium, and the ovoid mass excised from a labium minus proved to be choriocarcinoma. Chest x-rays were negative at this time, but 2 weeks later cough, fever to 103°, and delirium developed. She was given antibiotics and blood transfusions. A chest film revealed multiple bilateral nodular densities, and the patient was admitted to NIH on November 11, 1964. On admission, the uterus was enlarged, the ovaries were not palpable, and the HCG titer was $>$ 500,000 units. Chest x-rays confirmed previous findings. She received four courses of methotrexate therapy, followed by three courses of "triple therapy," and her hormone titer declined from a peak of 2 million units to the range of 2,000–5,000 units, then began to rise again. An additional course of actinomycin D alone followed by a fourth course of "triple therapy" proved unavailing. Pulmonary nodules persisted, increasing in size after transient, initial improvement. Thrombophlebitis developed in the arms and legs, extending into the inferior vena cava. Severe ulcerative pharyngitis and stomatitis further complicated the clinical picture. She died on March 19, 1965, 4 months after admission and 5 months after choriocarcinoma was diagnosed.

Autopsy (A-65–49) revealed the immediate cause of death to be laryngeal obstruction of a blood clot that had apparently formed from local mucosal ulceration of the hypopharynx and epiglottis. Metastatic choriocarcinoma was found in both lungs; the lesions were markedly necrotic with only small amounts of viable trophoblastic elements. Organizing thrombi occluded the inferior vena cava, both femoral veins, and the right subclavian vein. Evidence of drug toxicity was seen as severe fatty metamorphosis of the liver (FIGURE 186), acute necrotizing glossitis, stomatitis, pharyngitis, epiglottitis, esophagitis, and enteritis. Tiny foci of ectopic decidua were seen in the ovaries. [*Note:* In the absence of information regarding the nature of the antecedent gestation, this case is classified as choriocarinoma following pregnancy of undetermined type.]

GROUP II: Fatal Cases of Gestational Choriocarcinoma and Probable Choriocarcinoma, Not Autopsied

Case 45: N.G. (02–88–02), a 24-year-old gravida 3, para 2, had her last menstrual period in April, 1959, and passed a hydatidiform mole on September 4, 1959. Vaginal bleeding recurred a month later, and a curettage on October 5 yielded molar villi and sheets of proliferated trophoblast. The pregnancy test, which had been negative, became positive a week later. In January, she developed chest pain, and x-rays showed two nodules in the lungs. She was admitted to NIH on March 2, 1960. The HCG titer was > 1 million units, and the two pulmonary nodules had increased. After five courses of methotrexate, the titer had declined to less than 50 units, and the two chest nodules had disappeared. She was discharged "in remission" on May 13, 1960, but died suddenly at home, 2 days later, with signs of massive intracranial hemorrhage. No autopsy was performed.

A histopathological diagnosis of choriocarcinoma cannot be made, as the only morphologic material available could equally well be interpreted as chorioadenoma destruens. In the absence of an autopsy, one cannot exclude other forms of cerebrovascular accident as the cause of death, e.g., subarachnoid hemorrhage from an aneurysm of the circle of Willis. However, in view of the history, the presumptive diagnosis is choriocarcinoma metastatic to the brain.

Case 46: J.B. (02–30–53), a 19-year-old gravida 1, para 1, had her term delivery on October 22, 1958. Continuous vaginal bleeding required transfusions, and a curettage on November 17 yielded a few fragments of atypical trophoblast interpreted as "consistent with but not diagnostic of choriocarcinoma" (FIGURE 43). Chest x-rays disclosed secondary pulmonary deposits. She was admitted to NIH on January 15, 1959. The HCG titer was 4.5 million units. After six courses of methotrexate and six courses of vincaleukoblastine, the hormone titer had fallen to 20,000–50,000 units, and partial clearing of the pulmonary lesions was demonstrated roentgenographically. The patient was discharged on October 1, 1959, at her own request. The HCG titer on a specimen received on December 27 was 200,000 units. A subsequent communication from her family physician states that in March, 1960, she developed melena, hemoptysis, and a large abdominal mass; she died suddenly on March 18, 1960, 6 hours after admission to a hospital. No autopsy was performed; the duration of illness was 17 months.

Although histopathological material does not permit an unequivocal diagnosis of choriocarcinoma, the clinical context and subsequent course make this the most probable diagnosis.

Case 47: M.M. (01–76–04), a 36-year-old gravida 3, para 2, was curetted for an incomplete abortion in June, 1956. Only hemorrhagic decidua was recovered from the uterus. Vaginal spotting occurred in July and August, and profuse vaginal hemorrhage in September. A second curettage yielded only decidual tissue. In November, severe vaginal hemorrhage was treated by hysterectomy, and a diagnosis of choriocarcinoma was made (FIGURE 53). In January, 1957, she developed pain in the thoracic and lumbar spine followed by urinary incontinence. Over the next few months she lost 20 pounds, and when an x-ray disclosed a large mass in the chest (FIGURE 141), she was admitted to NIH on May 31, 1957. Shortly after admission, she collapsed and showed signs of massive intraperitoneal hemorrhage. She died on June 7, 1957, almost 1 year after the abortion. Permission for autopsy could not be obtained.

Case 48: V.B. (02–59–41), a 39-year-old divorced gravida 2, para 2, underwent dilatation and curettage for uterine bleeding on June 7, 1959, at which time a histopathological diagnosis of choriocarcinoma was made. A vaginal nodule excised at the same time contained syncytiotrophoblast. She denied pregnancy or any sexual intercourse for the past 4–5 years. She remained well until June, 1959, when a Friedman test was weakly positive, then unequivocally positive in July. She was admitted to NIH on August 3, 1959. The HCG titer was between 25,000 and 100,000 units. A chest x-ray showed a solitary nodule in the right lower lobe. The aorta was dilated, and this observation, coupled with other physical signs, led to a diagnosis of Marfan's syndrome. She received two courses of methotrexate, with decline of the hormone titer to 2,000 units and moderate reduction in the size of the intrapulmonic nodule. However, she signed out against advice, incompletely treated. Information received subsequently states that she died suddenly on November 6, 1959, following the abrupt onset of severe headache, coma, and convulsions. An autopsy was not performed.

Examination of histopathological materials from the uterine curettings showed solid masses of cytotrophoblast and syncytiotrophoblast. Sections of the uterine wall showed extensive invasion by typical choriocarcinoma. There was a decidual reaction in the endometrium. The tissue from the vaginal nodule was classified as a syncytial nodule. In the absence of a postmortem examination, there is no morphological confirmation of the probable cause of death as a cerebral metastasis with hemorrhage in an incompletely treated patient.

Case 49: A.L. (02–32–66), a 28-year-old gravida 8, para 4, aborta 3, mola 1, had her last abortion in January, 1956, last term delivery in January, 1957, and passed a hydatidiform mole in January, 1958 (FIGURES 13 & 14). Menses resumed normally to September, 1958, when menometrorrhagia developed and persisted to January 23, 1959, at which time a curettage was performed. A diagnosis of choriocarcinoma was made, and she was admitted to NIH on January 29, 1959; the HCG titer was between 500,000 and 2 million units. A large pelvic mass extending into the adnexa was palpated, and chest x-rays suggested bilateral secondary disease. She received three courses of methotrexate, and the hormone titer fell to about 200,000 units. A fourth course of methotrexate was begun, but the patient returned to her home against the advice of her physicians. She died on April 10, 1959. Permission for autopsy was refused, but the death certificate lists the cause of death as "choriocarcinoma in pelvis with metastases to both lungs," complicated by terminal bronchopneumonia.

This case is classified as "probable" choriocarcinoma because the only histopathological evidence on file at NIH consists of one slide of uterine curettings containing degenerating and necrotic tissue consistent with choriocarcinoma but not sufficiently well preserved to permit precise diagnosis. However, the course of the disease and the supporting endocrinological data leave little room for doubt.

Case 50: E.T. (02–45–33), a 28-year-old Negro gravida 3, para 1, aborta 1, mola 1, passed a hydatidiform mole in March, 1957, and a curettage was performed in April. The Friedman test was positive in May, and a hysterectomy was performed on May 24, 1957; the ovaries were not removed. She remained well for almost 2 years until April, 1959, when abdominal pain developed and a mass in the region of the right ovary was felt. The mass was removed at laparotomy on May 1, 1959, and diagnosed on pathological examination as choriocarcinoma. The patient was admitted to NIH on May 10, 1959; the HCG titer was between 2 million and 4 million units, and chest x-ray examination showed numerous large nodular densities in both lungs. She received six courses of methotrexate, with a decline of the hormone titer to 5,000–20,000 units and partial clearing of the chest x-rays. Then four courses of vincaleukoblastine were given, but the titer rose to the range of 20,000–50,000 units, and there was no further improvement in the chest films. She was discharged on pass for Christmas on December 15, 1959. Information received subsequently states that she died with signs and symptoms of intracranial hemorrhage on December 25, 1959, but no autopsy was performed.

GROUP III: Fatal Cases of Nongestational Choriocarcinoma, Autopsied

Case 57: B.L. (03–09–83), a 16-year-old nulligravida developed menometrorrhagia and abdominal swelling in December, 1959, and was first seen by her physician in March, 1960. Physical examination revealed a large abdominopelvic mass, and an excretory urogram showed mild hydronephrosis secondary to partial ureteral obstruction. A pregnancy test was negative. At laparotomy on March 24, 1960, a right ovarian mass was removed. Pathological examination yielded a diagnosis of embryonal carcinoma with focal trophoblastic elements (FIGURES 121–123). On April 4, the uterus, right fallopian tube, left ovary and tube, and vermiform appendix were removed. A small amount of residual tumor was found attached to the right tube. She remained well for 2 months, when a large abdominal mass was again palpable. She was admitted to NIH on July 19, 1960. The HCG titer was 5,000–20,000 units, and the chest x-ray was clear. She received two courses of methotrexate therapy, and the hormone titer fell to 2,000 units. Gas gangrene developed secondary to intestinal ulcers, and she died on August 14, 1960.

Autopsy (A-60–171) revealed choriocarcinoma metastatic to mesenteric and periaortic lymph nodes as well as necrotic tumor in the pelvic cul-de-sac. The small intestine was ulcerated and perforated with generalized intraperitoneal and retroperitoneal gas gangrene and massive hemoperitoneum.

Case 52: M.T. (01–72–49), a 32-year-old nulligravida, had never menstruated until November, 1956, when moderate vaginal spotting occurred. A frog test was positive in December, and she was considered pregnant. In January, 1957, she developed a cough and in February low-back pain and breast enlargement; a chest x-ray in March showed bilateral pulmonary nodules. Laparotomy at the end of March revealed a large tumor arising from the left ovary and extensive metastases in the liver. The uterus and left adnexal mass were removed. The right ovary was not found. Histopathological examination of the tumor disclosed a choriocarcinoma and dysgerminoma (FIGURES 125–127). X-Ray therapy to the chest and abdomen was given;

jaundice developed and progressed. She was admitted to NIH on April 29, 1957, and died 2 days later after receiving only two injections of methotrexate, a total dose of 50 mg; the duration of illness was 5 months.

Autopsy (A-57–86) showed choriocarcinoma metastatic to the liver (FIGURES 128 & 129), lungs (FIGURE 130), vagina (FIGURE 124), and diaphragm (FIGURES 131 & 132). No residual foci of disgerminoma were found. The endometrium in the hysterectomy specimen was in the secretory phase without decidual reaction. [*Note:* It is reasonable to infer that the neoplasm arose in the dysgenetic gonad.]

Case 53: A.B. (04–24–14), a 9-year-old girl, developed precocious puberty at about 7.5 years of age. After a few months, a left ovarian mass was detected and resected in April, 1962; it proved to be a combined teratocarcinoma and choriocarcinoma (FIGURES 133 & 134). She was first admitted to NIH in May, 1962; the HCG titer was between 200,000 and 500,000 units, and a chest x-ray showed bilateral nodular densities in the lungs. She received 16 courses of "triple therapy", combined methotrexate, chlorambucil, and actinomycin D with temporary improvement. On one occasion in January, 1963, the hormone titer was as low as 50 units, and the chest lesions showed diminution in number and size. However, by April, 1963, it was evident that she was resistent to therapy; the hormone titer had risen to admission levels, and pulmonary lesions were progressing. Signs of central nervous system involvement developed, and she died on May 12, 1963, 13 months after the diagnosis of choriocarcinoma.

Autopsy (A-63–103) disclosed choriocarcinoma metastatic to multiple sites in the cerebrum, meninges, lungs, liver, jejunum, kidneys, spleen, and thyroid gland. Terminal bronchopneumonia was present. The metastatic deposits were composed entirely of choriocarcinoma without other teratoid elements. The right ovary contained multiple small theca-lutein cysts (FIGURE 135), and there was hyperplasia of the ovarian hilar cells (FIGURE 136). The uterus and breasts were larger than expected for a child of 9 years; however, the endometrium showed no glandular secretion or decidual reaction (FIGURE 137). The breasts showed some proliferation of periductal stroma, but no glands had developed (FIGURES 249 & 250). A moderate amount of pubic hair was present, but axillary hair had not developed. The immediate cause of death was multiple cerebral metastases and terminal bronchopneumonia.

Case 54: B.H. (05–25–11), a 31-year-old Negro gravida 4, para 4, developed increase in abdominal girth, gastrointestinal distress, a weight loss of 10–15 pounds, and intermittent vaginal staining 5 years after the birth of her last child. An abdominopelvic mass was palpated to the right of the uterus. At laparotomy on September 30, 1963, abdominal carcinomatosis was discovered, secondary to a right ovarian tumor. Hysterectomy, bilateral salpingo-oophorectomy, and partial omentectomy were performed, but residual tumor nodules on the peritoneal surface of the liver and elsewhere were not removed. Histopathological examination of the tumor revealed it to be a combined disgerminoma and choriocarcinoma (FIGURES 138–140). A Hogben test 1 week after operation was positive. The patient was admitted to NIH on October 10, 1963. Urinary HCG titer was between 50,000 and 200,000 units; the chest x-ray was clear. Signs of intraperitoneal hemorrhage developed a few days after admission, and laparotomy was necessary to control bleeding from multiple sites of metastatic choriocarcinoma on the serosa of the liver and small intestine. Her postoperative course was complicated by acute renal shutdown. Three courses of methotrexate failed to lower the chorionic gonadotropin titer. X-Ray therapy to the abdomen was begun in December, 1963, but signs of peritonitis developed, complicated by agranulocytosis. Vaginal bleeding developed, followed by fever and a shaking chill. Signs of sepsis continued despite antibiotics, and she died on December 9, 1963, slightly more than 2 months after her first laparotomy.

Autopsy (A-63–236) disclosed choriocarcinoma metastatic to the liver, pancreas, spleen (FIGURE 230), and small intestine, and extensive nodular deposits on peritoneal surface. The secondary deposits were composed entirely of trophoblastic tissue without any disgerminomatous elements; the pattern of trophoblastic growth was curiously unlike that customarily seen in gestational choriocarcinoma. There were no metastases in the lungs or brain. The cause of death was massive necrotizing enteritis secondary to *Clostridium perfringens* infection, colonies of which were seen in the lungs (FIGURE 272), liver, and retroperitoneal tissue. Extensive growth of *Clostridium perfringens* was found in the vaginal mucosa, which may have served as a portal of entry; however, ulcerated devitalized deposits of choriocarcinoma in the submucosa of the small intestine cannot be excluded as an alternative portal. Toxic changes were seen in the kidneys, and focal ischemic lesions were noted in the myocardium.

GROUP IV: Nonfatal Cases of Gestational Choriocarcinoma, Histologically Verified Following Term Delivery

Case 55: M.A. (02–45–84), a 31-year-old primigravida, had her term delivery on March 6, 1959. Intermittent postpartum bleeding continued, and a curettage on April 17 yielded syncytial tissue (FIGURE 39). Although this tissue was not diagnosed as choriocarcinoma, bleeding persisted, and a hysterectomy was performed on April 24; a vaginal nodule was also excised. She was admitted to NIH on May 14, 1959. Review of the microscopical sections established the presence of choriocarcinoma in the uterine curettings as well as in the uterine wall and the vagina. On admission, there was a large pelvic mass, left pleural effusion, and roentgenographically demonstrable nodules in both lungs. The HCG titer was between 5 million and 10 million units. She received five courses of methotrexate, complicated by an episode of serum hepatitis between the third and fourth courses. The hormone titer fell to 5,000 units, and the chest lesions regressed almost completely. She was discharged on September 23, 1959, 4 months after admission.

Without further treatment, the hormone titer declined to the level of 200–500 units on follow-up examination in November; at that time, a small mass was still felt in the pelvis and a rather questionable lesion was seen in the chest film. She was reported well and without roentgenographic or hormonal evidence of disease in August, 1964, 5.5 years after delivery.

Case 56: G.B. (01–23–62), a 24-year-old gravida 8, para 5, had her last term delivery on January 8, 1956, and continued to bleed postpartum. Curettage 3 weeks after delivery produced tissue diagnosed as choriocarcinoma. A chest x-ray showed bilateral nodular densities, and a Friedman test was positive. She was admitted to NIH on March 3, 1956. The uterus was enlarged, and the HCG gonadotropin titer was between 4 million and 5 million units. A chest x-ray confirmed the presence of bilateral pulmonary deposits. She received two courses of methotrexate; the hormone titer declined, and the uterus decreased in size, but uncontrollable uterine bleeding developed, necessitating hysterectomy and bilateral salpingo-oophorectomy on April 17. The uterus contained choriocarcinomatous tissue (FIGURE 58). Further courses of methotrexate were given, to a total of seven courses in all. The HCG titer fell to the level of 20–100 units, and the chest lesions cleared. She was discharged on September 6, 1956, 6 months after admission.

Reevaluation in March, 1957, showed no change in her status, but she was readmitted in July with symptoms suggesting peptic ulcer and the statement that two Friedman tests performed elsewhere had been reported positive. A single course of methotrexate was given. Urinary HCG titers and two Friedman tests were negative. Follow-up to July, 1969, revealed no evidence of recurrent disease, 13 years after delivery.

Case 57: M.L.B. (01–96–50), a 24-year-old gravida 2, para 1, passed a hydatidiform mole spontaneously in April, 1955, following which her uterus was curetted. Menses resumed, and three frog tests were negative. She had a term delivery in September, 1956; menses were normal postpartum until March, 1957, when the flow became irregular and menorrhagia developed. A curettage in August, 1957, yielded only decidua (FIGURE 75). Uterine bleeding persisted, and a nodule appeared in the vagina; in September, another curettage was performed and the vaginal nodule excised. Both specimens were unequivocally diagnosed as choriocarcinoma (FIGURES 27, 29, 87 & 88). A hysterectomy, bilateral salpingo-oophorectomy, and wide vaginal excision were performed on September 10, 1957 (FIGURES 25, 26, & 28). There was abundant residual choriocarcinoma in the uterus, and the ovaries showed multiple theca-lutein cysts (FIGURES 106 & 107). In October, the HCG titer was over 250,000 units, and the patient was admitted to NIH on October 25, 1957. The hormone titer was between 1 million and 2 million units; a chest x-ray was negative. She received five courses of methotrexate, and the titer fell to the level of 1,000–2,500 units; she was discharged on January 13, 1958. The HCG titer rose to 80,000 units in March, and she was readmitted from March 12 to May 10, 1958, during which time she received another three courses of methotrexate and the hormone titer again fell to 1,000–2,000 units. Her titer remained at this level or lower until January, 1959, when it rose slightly to 4,000 units. She was readmitted, given her ninth course of methotrexate, and discharged on February 9, 1959. Titers remained low for 6 months, then rose ot the 5,000–10,000 unit range in August. Her third admission was from August 16 to October 5, 1959, when she received a tenth course of methotrexate and a single course of vincaleukoblastine. Since that time, she was followed and remained in good health with normal urinary HCG titers through October, 1964, 8 years after delivery.

Case 58: L.E. (03–26–97), a 37-year-old gravida 7, para 5, had her last term delivery on August 6, 1960. Persistent profuse postpartum bleeding necessitated curettage on September 19, and a histopathological diagnosis of choriocarcinoma was made. Hysterectomy with right salpingo-oophorectomy was performed on September 23. She was admitted to NIH on October 31, 1960. The HCG titer was between 200,000 and 500,000 units, and a chest x-ray showed several small nodules in both lung fields. Examination of sections from the uterus confirmed the diagnosis of choriocarcinoma; sections of the right ovary could not be obtained. She received two courses of methotrexate; the hormone titer fell to normal, and the chest nodules disappeared. She was discharged on December 12, 1960. Follow-up chest films and urinary HCG titers remained negative through November, 1964, 4 years and 3 months after delivery.

Case 59: J.G. (02–10–98), a 25-year-old gravida 3, para 3, had her last term delivery on February 26, 1958. Delayed postpartum bleeding developed 2 weeks later, and a curettage on April 21 led to a histopathological diagnosis of choriocarcinoma. At hysterectomy and bilateral salpingo-oophorectomy, choriocarcinoma was found (FIGURES 46 & 47), invading the myometrium; she was treated with nitrogen mustard. There was no evidence of recurrence until August, 1958, when an Aschheim-Zondak test was reported positive. She was given one dose of methotrexate orally, possibly 10 mg, and admitted to NIH on August 20, 1958. The chest x-ray was negative, and the HCG titer was 200–300 units. There being no evidence of local or metastatic disease, chemotherapy was withheld. The patient was followed and continued to have negative chest films and urinary HCG titers through January, 1969, almost 11 years after delivery. [*Note:* In view of the minimal chemotherapy given, this is listed as an untreated case, possibly adequately treated by hysterectomy alone.]

Case 60: F.G. (02–74–56), a 19-year-old gravida 4, para 4, had her last term delivery on August 4, 1959. The puerperium was normal for 3.5 weeks, when vaginal oozing developed; a curettage yielded only secretory endometrium, and a chest x-ray was negative. Shortly thereafter, a frog test for pregnancy was positive. An ischiorectal mass developed; incision and drainage of this fluctuant mass yielded friable tissue diagnosed microscopically as choriocarcinoma. At hysterectomy on October 19, 1959, choriocarcinoma was found in the uterus (FIGURE 62). A chest x-ray in November showed multiple bilateral nodules, and she was admitted to NIH on November 16, 1959. The HCG titer was between 500,000 and 2 million units; a chest x-ray confirmed the presence of secondary deposits in the lungs. She received three courses of methotrexate, and the hormone titer fell to the level of 200–500 units and the chest lesions disappeared. She was discharged on January 12, 1960, and showed no hormonal or roentgenographic evidence of disease to the time of her last follow-up examination in November, 1963, 4 years and 3 months after delivery.

Case 61: B.H. (02–73–75), a 34-year-old gravida 4, para 3, had her last term delivery on August 3, 1959. She continued to bleed moderately, and a curettage on October 13 yielded tissue diagnosed on microscopical examination as choriocarcinoma. Hysterectomy with bilateral salpingo-oophorectomy was performed a few days later; the uterus contained invasive choriocarcinoma. A chest x-ray at this time was negative, but 3 weeks later showed several nodules in both lung fields. The HCG titer was between 25,000 and 50,000 units. She was admitted to NIH on November 10, 1959; the hormonal and roentgenographic observations were confirmed, and she was treated with three courses of methotrexate. The hormone titer declined to 200–500 units, and the chest lesions regressed. She was discharged on December 24, 1959, but was readmitted for one more course of methotrexate on January 19, 1960, when the HCG titer rose to 1,000 units. She was discharged on January 31, 1960, and showed no endocrine or roentgenographic evidence of recurrent disease to the time of her last follow-up examination in January, 1965.

Case 62: F.R. (03–31–28), a 28-year-old gravida 2, para 2, had her second term delivery on September 14, 1960. Postpartum bleeding continued intermittently for 6 weeks, when curettage yielded tissue diagnosed microscopically as choriocarcinoma. Uterine bleeding continued, and a 10-pound weight loss was reported. The HCG titer was between 200,000 and 500,000 units, and a chest x-ray was clear. She was admitted to NIH on November 29, 1960; the hormone titer was between 2 million and 5 million units. Severe vaginal bleeding necessitated hysterectomy on December 1, 1960, but the ovaries were not removed; the uterus contained invasive choriocarcinoma. She received two courses of methotrexate, and the HCG titer fell to 200 units, then to 20–50 units. She was discharged on January 20, 1961, and has showed no endocrine or roentgenographic evidence of recurrence to the time of her last follow-up examination in November, 1964.

Case 63: E.S. (02–62–80), a 27-year-old gravida 2, para 2, had her second term delivery on June 4, 1959. Heavy postpartum spotting was noted for 4 weeks, but remitted. She was considered normal at the 6-week postpartum visit, but two weeks later began to bleed copiously and pass clots. Curettage on August 17, 1959, produced tissue diagnosed microscopically as choriocarcinoma, and she was admitted to NIH on August 28 with an enlarged uterus, a nodular density in the right lower lobe, and an HCG titer between 100,000 and 500,000 units. Hysterectomy was performed on September 2, but the ovaries were not removed. Pathological examination of the uterus showed invasive choriocarcinoma (FIGURE 20); the endometrium was in the secretory phase (FIGURE 71) with no decidual reaction. After one course of methotrexate, the hormone titer fell to the level of 200–500 units, and regressive changes were demonstrable in the chest nodule. Further chemotherapy was withheld, and the HCG titer declined to 50–200 units; the chest nodule disappeared. She was discharged on October 30, 1959. Hormone titers and chest films continued negative through August, 1969, more than 10 years after delivery.

Case 64: C. McE. (03–33–89), a 29-year-old primigravida, had her term delivery on October 20, 1960. Postpartum spotting continued for 3 to 4 weeks, then was followed by profuse bleeding. Curettage on November 18 yielded tissue diagnosed microscopically as choriocarcinoma (FIGURES 40–42). Uterine bleeding continued, and a second curettage was performed, yielding similar tissue. A frog test was negative on December 8, and she was admitted to NIH on December 19, 1960. The HCG titer was between 2 million and 5 million units, and a chest x-ray was negative. Mild thyrotoxicosis was diagnosed (PBI, 15.8 μg; I^{131} uptake, 54%). She received three courses of methotrexate; the hormone titer fell to 20–50 units, and the tests of thyroid function returned to normal values. She was discharged on April 25, 1961, and remained in good health with negative urinary hormone titers until she became pregnant again in March, 1964. Because of unexpected antepartum hemorrhage, delivery was by cesarean section, and this was followed by a hysterectomy, 4 years after her first delivery.

Case 65: B.S. (03–34–58), a 22-year-old gravida 3, para 3, had her last term delivery on October 11, 1960. The puerperium was normal until December 8, when a sudden episode of brisk vaginal bleeding caused her to lose consciousness. Curettage that day yielded tissue diagnostic of choriocarcinoma, and a hysterectomy with bilateral salpingo-oophorectomy was perfomed on December 13. A chest x-ray at the time showed a solitary nodule, but 3 weeks later a second film showed multiple nodules in both lung fields. She was admitted to NIH on December 20, 1960, with pleuritic chest pain. The HCG titer was between 500,000 and 2 million units, and review of the pathological material confirmed the diagnosis of invasive choriocarcinoma. She received three courses of methotrexate, and the hormone titer fell to between 2,000 and 5,000 units, with some clearing of the chest film. However, three more courses of methotrexate failed to produce further change, and two courses of actinomycin D were given. Following this therapy, the HCG titer fell to 200–500 units, and the chest lesions disappeared. Follow-up to January, 1965, showed no evidence of recurrent disease, 4 years and 3 months after delivery.

Case 66: C.W. (02–20–43), a 21-year-old primigravida, delivered an hydropic infant after 37 weeks of gestation on August 3, 1958. She developed persistent postpartum vaginal bleeding, and curettages on September 9 and September 28 yielded tissue diagnosed as choriocarcinoma on microscopical examination (FIGURE 38). Hysterectomy and bilateral salpingo-oophorectomy on October 17 showed invasive choriocarcinoma in the uterus; a preoperative HCG titer was reported as between 11,000 and 20,000 units. The ovaries (FIGURE 101) showed cystic follicles lined up beneath the tunica albuginea. The follicles were surrounded by mantles of luteinized theca-interna. She was admitted to NIH on October 24, 1958; a chest x-ray showed multiple bilateral secondary nodules, and the HCG titer was about 2 million units. She received six courses of methotrexate, with complete regression of the chest lesions and a decline in hormone titer to 2,000 units. She was discharged on February 9, 1959, in remission, but was readmitted on April 19, 1959, in relapse, with an HCG titer of 25,000 units and the appearance of a new nodule in the chest film. Two additional courses of methotrexate were given, and the hormone titer declined to 500–2,000 units, but a third course did not alter her status. After she was given one course of vincaleukoblastine, the hormone titer fell to 200 units and the chest nodule disappeared. She was discharged on July 25, 1959, in remission, but was readmitted on August 24 because the hormone titer has risen to between 2,000 and 5,000 units. A second course of vincaleukoblastine succeeded in lowering the titer to 200 units, and she was discharged on September 24, 1959. Follow-up observations to September, 1964, showed no endocrine or roentgenographic evidence of recurrence.

Case 67: V.B. (04–36–45), a 23-year-old gravida 7, para 7, delivered a female infant at term on April 8, 1962. Intermittent vaginal bleeding persisted until June 18, 10 weeks postpartum, when a syncopal episode led to hospitalization. Curettage the next day yielded tissue diagnosed microscopically as choriocarcinoma. Bleeding recurred on July 3, and she was admitted to NIH on July 4, 1962. The HCG titer was between 500,000 and 2 million units, and a chest x-ray showed no evidence of secondary deposits. A few hours after entry she went into shock from acute vaginal hemorrhage. One week later, after supportive therapy, a hysterectomy, bilateral salpingo-oophorectomy, appendectomy, cholecystectomy, and biopsy of a liver nodule were performed. The specimen showed choriocarcinoma superficially invading the myometrium (FIGURES 48–50), theca-lutein cysts of both ovaries, and chronic cholecystitis. No tumor was found in the liver nodule. Following surgery, the hormone titer fell to the level of 2,000–5,000 units. After two courses of actinomycin-D, the titer declined to the level of 500–2,000 units, and she was discharged on September 18, 1962, 5 months after delivery. The HCG level was in the range of 200–500 units or as low as 50–200 units through her last follow-up examination August 1964, at which time the patient was considered to have been in remission for 25 months.

Case 68: M.R. (03–66–49), a 31-year-old gravida 8, para 7, aborta 1, delivered a stillborn infant at term on May 22, 1961. Vaginal spotting persisted, and hormone medication was given for a few days. However, spotting was not controlled, and a curettage was performed on June 30. A histopathological diagnosis of choriocarcinoma was made, and the patient was admitted to NIH on July 9, 1961. The HCG titer was between 20,000 and 50,000 units; a chest x-ray showed four discrete nodules in the right lung field. She received four courses of methotrexate with partial remission, then three courses of actinomycin D. The pulmonary nodules cleared, and the hormone titer fell to the range of 200–500 units, then 10–15 units. She was discharged in remission on November 1, 1961, 5 months after delivery and 4 months after choriocarcinoma was diagnosed. Chest films and repeated hormone titers remained normal through January, 1965, 44 months after delivery.

Case 69: M.B. (03–59–47), a 22-year-old gravida 3, para 3, mola 1, delivered a male infant at term in July, 1960. Postpartum spotting and bleeding were continuous to December, when a curettage was performed and yielded "partially necrotic decidual tissue." Bleeding continued, and she was treated with hormone pills; Vaginal bleeding persisted, and the uterus was enlarged in February, but a pregnancy test was reported positive and a scheduled recurettage was postponed to observe the outcome of the suspected intrauterine pregnancy. In May, the patient developed a bullous rash diagnosed as erythema multiforme and treated with methylprednisolone. Bleeding persisted, and a second curettage was finally performed on May 24, 1961; choriocarcinoma was diagnosed on microscopical examination of the curettings. A chest film on June 5 showed multiple bilateral nodular densities; she was admitted to NIH on June 6, 1961. The HCG titer was 2 million units, and the chest x-ray contained innumerable nodules. The BMR was 52; PBI, 16.2 μg; and I^{131} uptake, 72.5%. She received five courses of methotrexate with almost complete regression of the pulmonary lesions, but the hormone titer declined only to the range of 20,000–50,000 units. She then received five courses of actinomycin D with decline of the titer to the level of 200–500 units. Tests of thyroid function returned to normal, concomitant with the regression of choriocarinomca. She was discharged over Christmas with persistent disease, and readmitted for hysterectomy on January 3, 1962. The hormone titer had risen to 5,000 units, and one additional course of methotrexate was given before hysterectomy with bilateral salpingo-oophorectomy on January 26. Following the operation, the titer declined to the range of 50–200 units, and she was discharged in remission on February 19, 1962, 19 months after delivery and 9 months after diagnosis. She was followed and remained in remission through September, 1964, 31 months after discharge.

Examination of the hysterectomy specimen (S-62–259) showed choriocarcinoma infiltrating the uterus, with extensive necrosis of the tumor. The ovaries showed some cystically dilated follicles and a persistent corpus luteum, but there were no theca-lutein cysts or stromal luteinization. A minute focus of ectopic decidua was present.

Case 70: L.D. (03–42–10), a 17-year-old gravida 1, para 1, had a term delivery on May 27, 1960. Postpartum bleeding persisted from July through January, 1961. During this time, she was treated with progesterone and cyclic norethynodrel. Dilatation and curettage on January 25, 1961, led to a diagnosis of choriocarcinoma based on microscopical examination of the curettings. Urinary assay for HCG was positive at 1:5,000 but negative at 1:10,000; a chest x-ray was negative. She was admitted to NIH on February 16, 1961, at which time the hormone titer was 2 million units. She received three courses of methotrexate with a decline in the hormone titer to 5,000 units, then six courses of actinomycin D without further effect. Combined treatment with chlorambucil and actinomycin D was begun in July, 1961, but the hormone titer rose to the range of 20,000–50,000 units. After hysterectomy and bilateral salpingo-oophorectomy on August 16, her subsequent titers were in the range of 200–500 units. She was discharged in remission on September 29, 1961, 16 months after delivery and 9 months after diagnosis, and was followed and remained in remission through February, 1965.

Pathological examination of the uterus revealed a small nodule of viable choriocarcinoma in the myometrium. The ovaries showed a few small theca-lutein cysts. [*Note:* The patient never had a positive chest film.]

Case 71: M.H. (03–42–70), a 16-year-old gravida 1, para 1, had a term delivery on September 26, 1960. Two episodes of abrupt vaginal bleeding occurred in November, and on November 24 a curettage was performed which was interpreted as "syncytial endometritis." She remained well until January 2, 1961, when spotting occurred, and on January 8 had a profuse hemorrhage. A second curettage on January 26 was interpreted as "atypical trophoblastic tissue consistent with choriocarcinoma." Review of these sections at NIH gave an unequivocal diagnosis of choriocarcinoma. A chest x-ray and a Friedman test on February 1 were both negative. However, an HCG assay on February 21 was positive at 2,000 units and negative at 5,000 units; she was admitted to NIH on February 22, 1961. After one course of methotrexate therapy, the hormone titer declined to the range of 50–200 units, and she was discharged in remission on March 28, 1961, 6 months after delivery. She was followed and remained in remission, with hormone titers in the 10–50 unit range and negative chest films, through April, 1965, 4.5 years after delivery.

Case 72: M.D. (03–40–98), a 28-year-old Negro gravida 1, para 1, had a term delivery in August, 1960. Intermittent vaginal spotting with intervals of heavier bleeding persisted until November, when a curettage yielded tissue diagnosed as "probable" choriocarcinoma. A pregnancy test was positive at that time and 1 month later, but no further surgery or specific treatment was instituted. In January, 1961, chest pain, fever, and a pulmonary infiltrate led to a diagnosis of "pneumopleuritis," which subsided after antibiotic therapy. Intermittent bleeding had persisted, and on January 21, 1961, a second curettage yielded an unequivocal histopathological diagnosis of choriocarcinoma. She was admitted to NIH on February 9, 1961. The HCG titer was between 2 million and 5 million units; chest x-rays showed no secondary deposits. She received three courses of methotrexate, and the hormone titer fell to borderline-positive at 200 units. She was discharged in remission on April 6, 1961; however, later that month and again in May the titer rose to 1,000 units, and she complained of lower abdominal pain. She was readmitted on May 21, 1961, received two more courses of methotrexate with a decline of the titer to 200 units, and was discharged on June 29, 1961, in remission. She was admitted for a third time on July 10 with a titer positive between 2,000 and 5,000 units. She received two more courses of methotrexate, then three courses of actinomycin D, and was discharged on October 13, 1961, with a titer of 50–200 units. Her fourth and final admission on January 23, 1962, was again occasioned by a rise in the hormone titer to the range of 5,000–20,000 units. After three more courses of actinomycin D, a hysterectomy with bilateral salpingo-oophorectomy was performed on March 12, 1962; the uterus contained a 3.5-cm mass superficially adherent to the wall, invading the myometrium no more deeply than 2 mm. Microscopical examination showed choriocarcinoma, with a decidual reaction in the uterine mucosa around the zone of attachment. The ovaries were only slightly enlarged, and contained theca-lutein cysts. Within a few days of the operation the HCG titer had declined to 200 units, and she was discharged on April 3, 1962, in remission, 19 months after delivery. She was followed and remained in good health, without evidence of elevated HCG titers, through June, 1964, almost 4 years after delivery.

Case 73: C.S. (04–09–44), a 25-year-old gravida 4, para 4, had a term delivery on November 26, 1961. During the first 6 weeks of the puerperium, she had episodic vaginal bleeding and lost weight. At her 6-week postpartum visit on January 10, 1962, a 1-cm swelling was noted at the hymeneal ring; it resembled a hematoma, and sitz baths were prescribed. She had recurrent severe vaginal bleeding 10 days later, and the "hematoma" was larger; on January 31, 1962, the vaginal nodule was excised, and a histopathological diagnosis of choriocarcinoma was returned. In February, the urinary HCG assay was positive at 1:3,000. On February 13, a new vaginal nodule was noted; she was admitted to NIH on February 26, 1962. The HCG titer was between 500,000 and 2 million units; the chest x-ray was free of nodules. The vaginal nodule was bleeding actively, and local excision was performed the day after entry to control bleeding. Microscopical examination showed metatastic choriocarcinoma. She received two courses of methotrexate, and the hormone titer fell to the level of 200 units. She was discharged in remission, with a hormone titer of 10–50 units, maintained through January, 1965, more than 3 years after delivery.

Following Hydatidiform Mole

Case 74: A.C. (02–50–15), a 31-year-old gravida 2, para 1, was curetted of a hydatidiform mole in April, 1958. She had had a thyroidectomy in 1950 for follicular carcinoma of the thyroid gland with metastases to regional lymph nodes, and was treated subsequently with radioactive iodine; there had been no recurrence. Her first pregnancy resulted in the term delivery of a normal infant in 1955. Following evacuation of the mole, the pregnancy test became negative, but intermittent vaginal bleeding led to a curettage in October, 1958, 6 months later. The curettings showed a late secretory endometrium with a decidual reaction in the stroma; small fragments of cytotrophoblast was identified, and a ghost chorionic villus was also seen, but no definite diagnosis could be established. Menses continued to be irregular for 5 months, and a second curettage was performed in March, 1959, 11 months after evacuation of the mole. The curettings showed scattered small clumps of trophoblastic elements, chiefly cytotrophoblast, but no chorionic villi. The pregnancy test was positive at this time. Total abdominal hysterectomy was performed on March 27, 1959, but the ovaries were not removed; the uterus showed invasive choriocarcinoma. Chest films were negative. Quantitative Aschheim-Zondek tests 3 and 6 weeks postoperatively gave titers of between 5,000 and 50,000 units. Chest films continued to be negative. The patient was admitted to NIH on June 9, 1959. The HCG titer was between 200 and 500 units, and a chest x-ray showed a single small nodule in the left lower lung field. She was treated with one course of methotrexate, and the chest lesion became smaller, but the hormone titer remained unchanged. She was discharged on July 17, 1959. On readmission on September 17, 1959, the hormone titer was between 50 and 200 units and the chest film was negative. Follow-up through July, 1964, showed no roentgenographic or endocrine evidence of disease, over 6 years after the mole was removed.

Case 75: J.E. (00–83–68), a 21-year-old primigravida, was curetted of a hydatidiform mole on July 20, 1956. Pregnancy tests 1 and 3 months later were negative, but irregular vaginal bleeding persisted. Curettage on December 20, 1956, 5 months after the mole, yielded trophoblastic tissue that was interpreted, at the time, as "probably retention of an invasive mole rather than choriocarcinoma." The patient missed her period in January, 1957, and was thought to be pregnant again. Scant vaginal bleeding appeared in February, at which time the uterus was slightly enlarged and the right ovary was larger than before. Two frog pregnancy tests were positive. Intermittent vaginal bleeding accompanied by nausea and vomiting persisted, but the uterus failed to enlarge. Symptoms continued for 5 months until July, 1957, when a curettage yielded sheets of trophoblastic tissue diagnosed as "either invasive mole or choriocarcinoma." A hysterectomy with bilateral salpingo-oophorectomy was performed on July 9, 1957; the uterus contained an invasive choriocarcinoma. Following the operation, she developed intermittent chest pain, low-grade fever, and persistent cough. Frog pregnancy tests were positive 2, 3, and 6 months postoperatively. A chest x-ray in February, 1958, showed an ill-defined infiltrate in the left lower lobe, and the patient was admitted to NIH on February 27, 1958. The HCG titer was between 500,000 and 1 million units. After four courses of methotrexate, the titer declined to between 500 and 1,000 units, and she was discharged on May 14, 1958, but re-admitted on June 16, 1958, with a hormone titer of 6,000 units. Two further courses of methotrexate produced a decline in the titer to 1,000 units, and the questionable lesion in the chest film disappeared by the time of her discharge on August 2, 1958. She was admitted for a third time on October 5, 1958, with a hormone titer of 10,000 units, received three further courses of methotrexate (nine courses in all) followed by a fall in the titer to between 200 and 500 units, and was discharged on November 18, 1958. There was no hormonal or roentgenographic evidence of recurrent disease through February, 1965, 8.5 years after the mole was removed.

Case 76: V.F. (02–01–75), a 22-year-old gravida 2, para 0, had a spontaneous abortion in March, 1956, then a hydatidiform mole evacuated by hysterotomy in October, 1956. Pregnancy tests were negative after the mole was evacuated, but vaginal bleeding developed in February, 1957, necessitating a hysterectomy and bilateral salpingo-oophorectomy on February 11, 1957. The uterus contained a choriocarinoma invading the superficial myometrium and subjacent blood vessels (FIGURES 65 & 66). The ovaries showed luteinization in the stroma, especially around atretic follicles. One week after hysterectomy, a chest x-ray was negative, but an Aschheim-Zondak test was positive. Bilateral nodules appeared in a chest film taken 7 weeks postoperatively, and she was treated with nitrogen mustard. Vaginal nodules appeared in July, 1957, and she received pelvic irradiation, following which the vaginal lesions regressed. Although a chest film in October, 1957, was negative, she complained of chest discomfort in November, had some difficulty in focusing her eyes, and the Aschheim-Zondak test was positive. She was admitted to NIH on December 10, 1957; The HCG titer was 250,000 units, and the chest x-ray was negative. After five courses of methotrexate therapy, the hormone titer had declined to 100 units, and she was discharged on April 3, 1958. Apart from menopausal symptoms, she remained well until March, 1960, when the HCG titer was reported as between 2,000 and 5,000 units. She was readmitted and received one course of methotrexate, the hormone titer falling to normal, and was discharged on April 20, 1960. Follow-up studies through January, 1969, showed no hormonal or radiological evidence of tumor, over 12 years after the mole was removed.

Case 77: V.H. (03–33–38), a 24-year-old gravida 2, para 1, was evacuated of a hydatidiform mole (FIGURES 15 & 16) by hysterotomy on June 29, 1960. Intermittent bleeding persisted, but Hogben tests remained negative to October, when a positive report was obtained. Curettage on October 10, 1960, yielded tissue diagnostic of choriocarcinoma, and a total abdominal hysterectomy was performed 3 days later; the uterus contained a large choriocarcinoma infiltrating widely and deeply (FIGURE 17), almost to the serosa. She was asymptomatic for a month, then developed chest pain and was admitted to NIH on December 12, 1960. Multiple nodules were seen in both lung fields (FIGURE 142) on chest x-ray, but the HCG titer was only between 200 and 500 units. After four courses of methotrexate, the chest lesions had almost entirely disappeared, and the hormone titer was between 50 and 200 units. She was discharged on February 10, 1961. Chest films over the next few months revealed gradual disappearance of all lesions (FIGURE 143), and she remained free of radiological or hormonal evidence of persistent or recurrent disease through January, 1969, 8.5 years after the mole was removed.

Case 78: N.L. (02–19–24), a 25-year-old gravida 2, para 1, was curetted of a hydatidiform mole in August, 1957. Menses resumed normally, and the patient was well until July, 1958, when amenorrhea developed. Vaginal bleeding occurred in October, 1958, and a vaginal nodule was found and excised. It was diagnosed as metastatic choriocarcinoma; she was admitted to NIH on October 17, 1958. The HCG titer was between 100,000 and 500,000 units, and a chest x-ray showed secondary nodules in both lungs. A repeat biopsy of the vaginal nodule showed metastatic choriocarcinoma, and 3,000 r of x-irradiation was given to the vaginal area to control bleeding. She received four courses of methotrexate, and the hormone titer fell to between 2,000 and 5,000 units. Her clinical course was complicated by serum hepatitis and a vesicovaginal fistula. She was discharged briefly and readmitted to receive two more courses of methotrexate. Following the sixth course, the vesicovaginal fistula healed, and the hormone titer fell to 100–200 units. The chest nodules had almost completely regressed, and she was discharged, in remission, on June 29, 1959. Follow-up observations through January, 1965, showed no endocrine or radiological evidence of disease, 7.5 years after the mole was removed.

Case 79: T.O. (02–27–29), a 17-year-old primigravida, was curetted of a hydatidiform mole in May, 1958. An episode of vaginal bleeding led to a curettage 2 months later which was reported as "negative," but bleeding persisted intermittently, and a second curettage in October, 1958, yielded tissue diagnosed as "trophoblastic tumor." Hysterectomy and bilateral salpingo-oophorectomy on October 13, 1958, showed choriocarcinoma infiltrating the uterus. Following operation, she remained asymptomatic, but was admitted to NIH on December 15, 1958, for evaluation. The chest x-ray was negative, and the HCG titer was between 200 and 500 units. She was discharged on January 5, 1959, untreated and with no evidence of active disease. A repeat HCG titer in June, 1959, was between 20 and 50 units. When last examined in November, 1964, she had no evidence of persistent trophoblastic disease, 6.5 years after the mole was removed. [*Note:* This is an example of choriocarcinoma adequately treated by hysterectomy without need for chemotherapy after operation.]

Case 80: L.P. (03–04–77), a 34-year-old gravida 3, para 2, had normal full-term deliveries in 1948 and 1951. One month after the second pregnancy, she had vaginal bleeding, and a curettage at that time was stated to have shown tissue compatible with a hydatidiform mole. During that year (1951–1952) she was curetted four times more, but no trophoblastic tissue was recovered; her chest x-ray and several Friedman tests were all reported negative. In 1955, a menstrual period was delayed for 2 weeks; this was followed by a normal period, after which she resumed cyclical menstruation at intervals of 40–45 days, instead of 30-day intervals as before. In October, 1959, her menstrual period lasted longer than usual. A chest x-ray showed a lesion in the left lower lobe, and a Friedman test was positive. Curettage did not recover trophoblast; hysterectomy was performed, but no tumor was found in the uterus. A small focus of atypical squamous cells was seen in the exocervix (FIGURE 82); the ovaries were not removed. The Friedman test remained positive, and a left lower lobectomy on February 2, 1960, showed metastatic choriocarcinoma (FIGURES 160 & 161). The Friedman test became negative a few days postoperatively, but was positive in March, negative in April, and positive again in May, when a chest film showed a questionable new lesion in the left lung. She was first admitted to NIH on June 20, 1960. The HCG titer was between 20,000 and 50,000 units; the chest x-ray was interpreted as negative. During three separate admissions to NIH, she received a total of ten courses of methotrexate, being discharged finally on May 19, 1961, with a hormone titer of 20–50 units. Follow-up studies showed no evidence of recurrent disease through November, 1964, 4 years and 9 months after lobectomy.

Case 81: A.R. (02–13–11), a 27-year-old gravida 3, para 2, passed a hydatidiform mole spontaneously on June 15, 1958, and was curetted for uterine bleeding on August 2 and August 5, 1958. The diagnosis at that time was "retained hydatidiform mole and syncytial endometritis." Severe bleeding recurred on September 3 and necessitated an emergency hysterectomy and right salpingo-oophorectomy; a mass in the right broad ligament could only be partially resected. The uterus showed invasive choriocarcinoma; she was admitted to NIH on September 20, 1958. The HCG titer was between 4 million and 6 million units, and the chest x-ray showed multiple large and small bilateral secondary pulmonary deposits. After five courses of methotrexate, the hormone titer fell to 200 units, and the chest film cleared. She was discharged on November 14, 1958. In February, 1959, the hormone titer was 10–50 units, and follow-up observations revealed no change through August, 1964, 6 years after the mole was passed.

Case 82: B.R. (04–50–16), a 37-year-old gravida 2, para 1, passed a hydatidiform mole in January, 1962, and was curetted. Vaginal bleeding began in March and grew progressively more severe. A second curettage on March 21 yielded tissue diagnosed microscopically as choriocarcinoma, and on March 26 a hysterectomy with bilateral salpingo-oophorectomy was performed. The specimen showed choriocarcinoma infiltrating the uterus; the ovaries contained theca-lutein cysts and a persistent corpus luteum of pregnancy (FIGURE 94). At this time, the HCG titer was 25,000 units.

Between April and August, urinary aliquots were sent to NIH for HCG assay; the level rose slowly from 200 units in April to over 2,000 units on August 13. A nodule was detected on a chest film, and the patient was admitted to NIH on August 31, 1962. The HCG titer was between 50,000 and 200,000 units, and a chest x-ray showed several well-circumscribed nodular densities in both lung fields. She received three courses of actinomycin D; the hormone titer declined to the range of 200–500 units, and the pulmonary nodules decreased in size. She was discharged on October 30, 1962, with persistent evidence of pulmonary nodules, but these slowly resolved and finally disappeared by May, 1963. Hormone titers and chest films remained normal and consistent with remission through March, 1965, more than 3 years after the mole was passed.

Case 83: C.O'G. (04–45–66), a 23-year-old primigravida, was curetted of a hydatidiform mole on March 1, 1962. The uterus did not involute satisfactorily, and vaginal bleeding continued; a frog test was negative. A second curettage on April 1 yielded retained hydatidiform villi and "active" trophoblast; a chest x-ray was clear. Menses did not resume, and in July she experienced sudden onset of profuse vaginal bleeding. A third curettage on July 16 yielded tissue diagnosed microscopically as choriocarcinoma. Severe vaginal bleeding persisted, requiring emergency hysterectomy and bilateral salpingo-oophorectomy on July 26. Pathological examination of this specimen showed infiltrating choriocarcinoma; sections of the ovaries could not be obtained for review. Chest x-rays, which had previously been negative, showed bilateral nodular infiltrates on August 7. Oral methotrexate therapy had been begun on August 3, and was continued until the patient was admitted to NIH on August 11, 1962. The HCG titer was between 50,000 and 200,000 units, and the chest film confirmed the presence of bilateral nodular densities. She received four courses of methotrexate; the hormone titer fell to about 1,000 units, and the chest lesions regressed completely. She was discharged on October 29, 1962, 8 months after the hydatidiform mole was first curetted. Follow-up studies showed continuing decline of the hormone titer to the range of 200–500 units, and remission was maintained through October, 1964, 2 years and 8 months after the mole.

Case 84: P.H. (03–52–16), a 35-year-old gravida 3, para 2, mola 1, was curetted of a hydatidiform mole on February 14, 1961. Microscopical examination of the mole showed "marked trophoblastic activity" (FIGURE 7). Vaginal spotting continued for 2 weeks after curettage; she then had a sudden profuse vaginal hemorrhage and was readmitted in shock on March 5. Curettage showed trophoblastic tissue without villi and was interpreted as choriocarcinoma (FIGURE 33); the endometrium was in the secretory phase (FIGURE 72). A Friedman test on serum was positive at 1:250; the chest film was clear. One week later, the Friedman test was positive at 1:1,000, and hysterectomy with bilateral salpingo-oophorectomy was performed on March 17, 1961. The uterus was invaded by choriocarcinoma (FIGURE 61) and the ovaries showed theca-lutein cysts. One month later, the chest film showed multiple secondary deposits and the Friedman test was strongly positive. She was admitted to NIH on April 21, 1961. The HCG titer was between 20,000 and 50,000 units, and a chest x-ray showed bilateral pulmonary nodules. Following three courses of methotrexate, the hormone titer fell to 50–200 units, and the chest film became clear. She was discharged on June 15, 1961, 4 months after evacuation of the mole, and remained in remission, on the basis of endocrinological and roentgenographic criteria, through January, 1965, almost 4 years after the mole was curetted.

Case 85: B.M. (03–62–09), a 28-year-old gravida 4, para 2, aborta 1, mola 1, underwent hysterotomy for evacuation of a hydatidiform mole on January 26, 1961. Scrapings from the attachment site showed atypical trophoblastic proliferation, with nests of cells in decidual sinuses. A frog test was positive 2 days after surgery but negative 3 weeks later. Vaginal bleeding developed in March, and a frog test was positive on March 23. Curettage yielded proliferating trophoblast and two molar villi; a diagnosis of retained hydatidiform mole was returned. The uterus involuted to normal size, and the frog test became negative. Bleeding recurred in mid-May, and the frog tests became positive. Hysterectomy with left oophorectomy was performed on May 23; the uterus was invaded by choriocarcinoma, and the ovary contained two luteinized cysts. Frog tests fluctuated from negative to positive; chest films showed no secondary lesions. The patient was admitted to NIH on June 15, 1961. The HCG titer was positive at 5,000 units and negative at 50,000 units; the chest x-ray showed diffuse secondary deposits. She received two courses of methotrexate, followed by clearing of the pulmonary lesions and decline of the hormone titer to 10–50 units. She was discharged in remission on August 9, 1961, 8 months after hysterotomy and 3 months after choriocarcinoma was diagnosed. She was followed and remained in remission with negative chest films and normal HCG titers through April, 1965, 4 years and 3 months after hysterotomy.

Case 86: S.T. (03–88–55), a 49-year-old gravida 7, para 7, underwent complete abdominal hysterectomy and unilateral salpingo-oophorectomy for hydatidiform mole on October 27, 1960. Pathological examination was said to have revealed a molar pregnancy with trophoblastic cells penetrating the uterine wall, but sections from this specimen were not available for review at NIH. Frog tests were negative through February, 1961. Late in June, she developed hemoptysis, and a chest x-ray showed two coin lesions in the right lung; a frog test was negative at this time. One of the coin lesions in the right lung was excised at thoractomy on July 3, 1961; the other was 6 cm in estimated size and could not be resected because of its location at the hilus, attached to and obstructing the azygos vein. Pathological examination of the excised nodule showed choriocarcinoma metastatic to lung. She was treated with seven courses of methotrexate between July and October, but the remaining pulmonary lesion gradually increased in size, and the HCG level did not fall below 500 units. She was admitted to NIH on October 20, 1961, with an HCG level of 20,000 units; a chest film showed the mass at the right hilum. She received four courses of actinomycin D; the chest lesion regressed, and the hormone titer fell to the level of 200–500 units. She was discharged in remission on December 21, 1961, 14 months after the hysterectomy for hydatidiform mole. Hormone titers were maintained at the 200–500 unit level and the chest film remained clear through her last follow-up in March, 1964, 3.5 years after her hysterectomy.

Following Abortion

Case 87: R.B. (01–80–71), a 24-year-old gravida 2, para 1, had a probable spontaneous abortion in October, 1956, followed by a curettage a few days later. Choriocarcinoma was diagnosed on pathological examination of the curettings, and hysterectomy was performed shortly thereafter; the uterus contained invasive choriocarcinoma. She remained asymptomatic until June, 1957, when she developed acute abdominal pain. Laparotomy showed a cyst of the left ovary which was resected, but the right ovary appeared normal and was not removed. Pathological examination of the left ovary revealed multiple follicular cysts. A few days later she began to bleed from a scalp lesion, which was excised; pathological examination revealed metastatic choriocarcinoma to the scalp (FIGURES 268, 269). She was admitted to NIH on July 3, 1957. The HCG titer was 2 million units, and a chest x-ray showed a nodular lesion in the apex of the right lung. Neurological signs were present, and an electroencephalogram was abnormal. She received four courses of methotrexate, with a fall of the hormone titer to 100 units, decrease in the size of the pulmonary nodule, remission of the neurological signs, and reversion of the electroencephalogram to a normal pattern. Follow-up studies through January, 1965, showed normal chest films and hormone titers never higher than 200 units. The patient was still free of disease, 8 years and 3 months after the abortion.

Case 88: A.C. (03–30–82), a 25-year-old Negro gravida 2, para 1, had a normal full-term delivery in 1955, and a spontaneous abortion in September, 1959, followed by curettage. The curettings contained a single focus of atypical trophoblast (FIGURE 45). Menses resumed normally to June, 1960, when vaginal bleeding developed. It persisted, and she was treated by a series of injections with a clinical diagnosis of threatened abortion until October, when the diagnosis was changed to "uterine fibroids." Hysterectomy with right salpingo-oophorectomy was performed on October 26, 1960; pathological examination of a soft tumor extending through the uterine wall into the right parametrium showed choriocarcinoma. A chest film postoperatively showed a patchy infiltrate in the right lower lobe, interpreted as pneumonitis; No hormone studies were done. She was admitted to NIH on November 26, 1960; The chest x-ray was negative, but the HCG titer was 5 million units. Following four courses of methotrexate, the hormone titer fell to 50–200 units, and the chest lesion cleared. Follow-up observations through December, 1964, disclosed no evidence of recurrent disease, 5 years and 3 months after the abortion.

Case 89: E.R. (02–81–69), a 26-year-old Negro gravida 5, para 3, aborta 2, had a curettage for incomplete abortion in July, 1959. At that time, "increased trophoblastic activity" was noted on pathological examination of the curettings; within a week of the curettage a chest x-ray and the HCG titer were both negative. In September, 2 months later, the uterus was not enlarged, and a chest film was again negative; the uterus was slightly enlarged 1 month later. She was next seen in January, 1960, for profuse vaginal bleeding; she had noted a lump in the vagina 2 weeks previously. Biopsy of the vaginal mass showed metastatic choriocarcinoma, and she was admitted to NIH on January 16, 1960. Vaginal bleeding could not be controlled, and a hysterectomy and partial colpectomy in continuity were performed on January 21, 1960. The uterus contained an invasive choriocarcinoma (FIGURE 60). The HCG titer on admission was between 500,000 and 2 million units; 1 week after operation, it had declined to between 50,000 and 200,000 units; 2 weeks after operation, it was between 20,000 and 50,000 units. A chest x-ray showed two small nodules in the right lung (FIGURE 144). Two courses of methotrexate therapy were given; the hormone titer fell to between 200 and 500 units, and the chest nodules disappeared. She was discharged on March 18, 1960, but readmitted on May 24 with a rise in the hormone titer to 20,000 units. Four more courses of methotrexate and three courses of vincaleukoblastine were complicated by hepatotoxicity and failed to produce more than transient effects on the hormone titer. She was discharged on December 16, 1960, with an elevated HCG titer. She was admitted for a third time on March 15, 1961, and given three courses of actinomycin D, with a fall in the hormone titer to the level of 50–200 units. The chest film was clear (FIGURE 145). She was discharged on May 24, 1961. Repeated follow-up observations through June, 1964, showed no evidence of recurrent disease, almost 5 years after the abortion.

Case 90: J.S. (06–46–42), a 46-year-old gravida 2, para 1, aborta 1, procured a criminal abortion in Cuba during January, 1959. She was asymptomatic until April, when vaginal bleeding occurred. Curettage yielded tissue diagnostic of choriocarcinoma; hysterectomy with bilateral salpingo-oophorectomy was performed promptly. The uterus was diffusely and deeply infiiltrated by choriocarcinoma (FIGURE 64), and she was admitted to NIH on May 18, 1959. The HCG titer was between 500,000 and 2 million units, and two small nodules were seen in the chest x-ray. After four courses of methotrexate, the hormone titer had fallen to the level of 200–500 units, and the chest film was clear. She was discharged on August 31, 1959. Follow-up observations through July, 1964, showed no hormonal or radiological evidence of recurrent disease, 5.5 years after the abortion.

Case 91: S.G. (02–31–24), a 16-year-old primigravida, had a spontaneous abortion in April, 1958, without medical supervision. Irregular vaginal bleeding persisted to September, but apparently normal menses occurred in October, November, and December. Profuse vaginal bleeding developed on January 6, 1959. A vaginal nodule (FIGURES 89 & 90) was excised, and curettage was performed 6 days later; both tissues were diagnostic of choriocarcinoma. A pregnancy test was positive, and a chest x-ray showed multiple bilateral secondary deposits. She was admitted to NIH on January 20, 1959; the HCG titer was between 100,000 and 200,000 units, and a chest x-ray confirmed prévious observations. She received four courses of methotrexate followed by a decline in the hormone titer to the level of 50–200 units and clearing of the chest film. She was discharged on March 21, 1959, but readmitted on July 31, 1959, because of an elevated HCG titer on a specimen sent in. On August 4, the titer was between 500,000 and 1 million units. Following two courses of methotrexate, she aborted a normal intrauterine pregnancy. There was no evidence of choriocarcinoma in the products of conception, and she was discharged on September 29, 1959. Follow-up observations through October, 1964, showed normal hormone titers and clear chest films, 6.5 years after the first abortion.

Case 92: A.P. (02–33–95), a 19-year-old gravida 2, para 1, was curetted for an incomplete abortion on September 24, 1958. One month later, uterine bleeding developed and a pelvic mass was palpated. Laparotomy revealed a tumor involving the uterus, ovaries, and appendix; a total abdominal hysterectomy with bilateral salpingo-oophorectomy was performed on November 20. Pathological examination showed choriocarcinoma invading the uterus (FIGURES 54, 55); sections of the ovaries were not submitted for examination. She was treated by pelvic irradiation and was relatively asymptomatic for 6 weeks, when cough and hemoptysis developed. A chest x-ray showed multiple bilateral nodular densities, and she was admitted to NIH on February 8, 1959. The HCG titer was between 100,000 and 500,000 units, and a chest film confirmed previous observations; a vaginal nodule was found on pelvic examination. Following one course of methotrexate, the hormone titer fell to the level of 200–500 units, and the chest lesions gradually cleared. Follow-up studies through November, 1964, over 6 years after the abortion, showed no endocrine or radiological evidence of recurrent disease.

Case 93: M.S. (01–94–22), a 21-year-old primigravida, developed vaginal bleeding in February, 1957, which required several curettages and multiple transfusions. The diagnosis was "spontaneous incomplete abortion," but histopathological documentation is lacking. She was admitted to a university hospital on April 19, 1957, where a pregnancy test was positive and curettage yielded tissue diagnostic of choriocarcinoma. Hysterectomy with bilateral salpingo-oophorectomy was performed 10 days after admission. The uterus contained invasive choriocarcinoma (FIGURE 57); sections of the ovaries were not reviewed at NIH. The HCG titer was positive at a dilution of 1–10 million, and a chest x-ray showed numerous scattered rounded densities in both lungs. A pituitary stalk section was performed on May 22, 1957; a chest film 3 weeks later showed some regression of pulmonary lesions. She was discharged on cortisone therapy, but her general status declined over the next 3 months, and she was admitted in debilitated condition, with multiple decubiti, to NIH on October 10, 1957. The chest films were clear, but the HCG titer was 100,000 units. She received one course of methotrexate and extensive local therapy to her decubiti. The hormone titer fell to the level of 200–500 units; the decubiti slowly healed, and cortisone was discontinued. She was discharged on March 26, 1958, in remission. Follow-up studies through November, 1964, showed normal hormone titers and clear chest films, 7 years and 9 months after the abortion.

Case 94: H.H. (04–37–27), a 39-year-old gravida 5, para 4, had a spontaneous abortion in May, 1959. Prior to this and for 1 year thereafter, her menses were always regular. Menstrual irregularity began in the summer of 1960, and daily spotting late in 1961; her breasts became tender and slightly swollen. In May, 1962, she developed intermittent, stabbing, right lower quadrant pain, and on June 11 consulted her physician, who found the uterus to be enlarged to within 3 cm of the umbilicus. Further enlargement was noted on June 25, and 2 days later, immediately after coitus, she experienced a sudden onset of pain in the abdomen and right shoulder, went into shock, and was hospitalized. At laparotomy, 2,000 cc of blood was found to have extravasated from a perforation in the right lower uterine segment; hysterectomy was performed; the ovaries were not removed. Pathological examination of the uterus showed infiltrating choriocarcinoma, and the patient was admitted to NIH on July 9, 1962. The HCG titer was $>$ 2 million units, and a chest x-ray showed scattered nodular densities in both lung fields. She received six courses of actinomycin D and four courses of methotrexate. The hormone titer fell to the level of 50–200 units, and the chest lesions cleared. She was discharged in remission on December 17, 1962, 6 months after choriocarcinoma was diagnosed. Hormone titers were maintained at the 50–200 units level, and chest films remained clear through January, 1965, more than 5.5 years since the abortion.

Case 95: I.D. (03–68–67), a 37-year-old gravida 2, aborta 2, had normal menses to November, 1960, when she had a painful period lasting 1 day. In mid-December, her period was unusually heavy, and she may have passed tissue. In February, 1961, she had an attack of severe lower abdominal pain, following which a rabbit test was positive for pregnancy. Vaginal spotting developed, but no more tissue was passed. On April 1, 1961, she had another attack of severe abdominal pain and profuse vaginal bleeding with shock. Cul-de-sac aspiration yielded bloody fluid, and a laparotomy disclosed 500–600 cc of blood and clot in the peritoneal cavity; a hemorrhagic mass was seen at one uterine cornu. The uterus, left tube and ovary, and appendix were removed. In June, she developed nausea, vomiting, and constipation; a tender mass was felt in the midline above the vaginal apex. Laparotomy revealed a 7-cm pelvic mass, adherent anteriorly to the peritoneum and posterior to the sigmoid and sigmoid mesentery; this mass and a cystic right ovary were removed. Microscopical examination of the uterus showed infiltration by choriocarcinoma; the pelvic mass was diagnosed as recurrent choriocarcinoma; the ovaries contained theca-lutein cysts. On admission to NIH on July 20, 1961, the HCG titer was between 50,000 and

500,000 units. A questionable small nodule was seen in the right upper lobe of a chest x-ray. She received three courses of methotrexate, following which the hormone titer declined to the range of 200–500 units and the questionable pulmonary nodule disappeared. She was discharged in remission on September 12, 1961, 5.5 months after choriocarcinoma was diagnosed. Hormone titers and chest x-rays remained normal through April, 1965, about 4.5 years after the last abortion.

Case 96: J.W. (04–29–26), a 26-year-old gravida 2, para 1, aborta 1, had a spontaneous abortion after 3 months of gestation in September 1960, associated with excessive bleeding and curettage, and requiring blood transfusion. Following this, her periods became irregular, with frequent intermenstrual spotting and menorrhagia; partial improvement was effected with cyclical norethynodrel medication. She thought she had a normal period in November, 1961, missed her period in December, had heavy vaginal bleeding with clots in January, and on norethynodrel had subjectively normal menses in February and March. She did not bleed on norethynodrel withdrawal as expected early in April, but bled spontaneously late in April. A mass was felt in the cul-de-sac on May 23, 1962, and she was hospitalized. A frog test was positive at 1:100 and negative at 1:1,000; a chest x-ray revealed multiple nodular densities. Curettage on May 26, 1962, yielded large amounts of necrotic tissue diagnosed microscopically as choriocarcinoma. Hysterectomy with right salpingo-oophorectomy was performed on May 29; The uterus was infiltrated by choriocarcinoma; sections of the right ovary were not transmitted for review. She was admitted to NIH on June 10, 1962, with an HCG titer between 2 million and 5 million units, and a chest x-ray showing extensive bilateral secondary deposits. She received four courses of methotrexate, and the hormone titer fell to the range of 200,000 units. She then received seven courses of actinomycin D, and the titer declined to about 200 units. By the time of discharge on December 15, 1962, the chest lesions had largely regressed. On subsequent readmissions for evaluation there was no further change in the chest films, and the residual small irregular densities could not be distinguished from focal fibrosis. Hormone titers remained consistently in the range of 10–50 units through December, 1969, 9 years and 3 months after the abortion.

GROUP V: Nonfatal Cases of Probable Gestational Choriocarcinoma

Case 97: A.A. (01–62–39), a 29-year-old primigravida, was curetted to evacuate a hydatidiform mole on November 25, 1954. Aschheim-Zondak (A-Z) tests continued positive until January 6, 1955, and a second curettage on January 19 showed a decidual reaction in the endometrium. Menses were scanty and irregular, not resuming normal character until June, 1955. The A-Z tests continued to be positive until January, 1956, and were then negative until September, 1956, when a positive A-Z test was interpreted as indicating a new pregnancy. She complained of abdominal pain in December, 1956, and examination disclosed bilateral ovarian masses. At laparotomy on January 5, 1957, the uterus was enlarged to the size of a 3-month gestation; wedge biopsies from both ovaries showed multiple theca-lutein cysts and stromal luteinization. Shortly thereafter, she developed cough, chills, and fever, and a chest x-ray showed multiple large and small nodular densities in both lung fields; another A-Z test was positive. She had lost 20 pounds and appeared cachectic, and was admitted to NIH on February 7, 1957. The HCG titer was between 10 million and 12 million units, and a chest x-ray confirmed the presence of extensive secondary pulmonary disease. After six courses of methotrexate, the hormone titer fell to 1,000 units. Hyperthyroidism was treated with methimazole. At hysterectomy and bilateral salpingo-oophorectomy on May 8, 1957, the uterus contained a large mass of necrotic tissue lying in its wall and impinging on the endometrial surface. On examination of multiple sections, no viable trophoblast was seen; the mass was composed of necrotic tissue, fibrin, and amorphous debris (FIGURES 30–32). One ovary contained a luteinized structure in which calcospherites were seen (FIGURE 110). She was discharged briefly on May 30, 1957, with the HCG titer at 5,000 units and residual pulmonary lesions that showed radiological evidence of regression. Between June, 1957, and April, 1960, she was readmitted to NIH on ten occasions with elevated hormone titers; during these admissions, she received at varying times a course of treatment with 6-mercaptopurine, 14 more courses with methotrexate, and four courses of vincaleukoblastine. The chest lesions became radiologically invisible by September, 1957, and the hormone titer finally leveled off at 500–1,000 units in May, 1960, and continued in the range of 50–200 units through October, 1964, almost 10 years after the original hydatidiform mole was removed.

This case is classified as "probable" choriocarcinoma because there has been no histopathological identification of any viable trophoblastic tissue since the original hydatidiform mole. The extremely elevated HCG titer, the positive chest x-rays, and the gravity of the patient's condition in January and February, 1957, support the presumptive diagnosis of choriocarcinoma; however, definitive histopathological proof is lacking, since the uterine tumor was destroyed by chemotherapy before hysterectomy.

Case 98: J.C. (01–26–29), a 23-year-old-gravida 2, para 1, was treated for a hydatidiform mole (FIGURE 11 & 12) by hysterotomy in August, 1952. She became pregnant again in December, 1953, and had a normal term delivery on August 8, 1954. Moderate menorrhagia appeared after delivery, but gynecological examination in January, 1955, disclosed no abnormalities. Menses were regular to September, 1955, followed by moderate menorrhagia to January, 1956. A so-called "cyst of the urethra" ruptured spontaneously with bleeding in February, 1956. From October, 1955, to March, 1956, she experienced episodes of cough and chest pain. In March, 1956, she had an episode of moderately severe hemoptysis, and a few days later vaginal hemorrhage with the passage of clots. She was admitted to a local hospital for curettage; the uterus was enlarged, and a Friedman test was positive, but the curettings showed only decidual tissue; a chest x-ray was negative. On March 24, 1956, she was readmitted because of nodular masses in the labia. A biopsy was interpreted as showing choriocarcinoma (FIGURES 34 & 35), and she was admitted to NIH on April 11, 1956. The HCG titer was between 200,000 and 400,000 units, and a chest x-ray showed bilateral pulmonary infiltration. A hemorrhagic, fungating mass had replaced much of the vulva and encroached on the perineum. Between April, 1956, and May, 1957, she received 17 courses of methotrexate; the chest films became clear by July, 1956, but the HCG titer, which declined promptly to between 10,000 and 20,000 units, did not finally become normal until after hysterectomy and bilateral salpingo-oophorectomy in April, 1957. As in case 97, the uterus contained a large mass of necrotic tissue in which multiple sections failed to reveal any viable trophoblastic tissue (FIGURES 36 & 37). The patient was followed and remained well and free from endocrine or roentgenographic evidence of trophoblastic disease through January, 1965, 19 years and 5 months following her last pregnancy.

Review of the biopsies for the mass involving the labia and perineum disclosed a hemorrhagic and necrotic neoplasm strongly suggestive of choriocarcinoma, but not sufficiently well preserved in histological appearance to permit a definitive diagnosis of choriocarcinoma on morphological grounds alone, unsupported by the clinical context. Therefore, this case is classified as "probable" choriocarcinoma despite the strong support for this diagnosis by the clinical course, HCG titers, and chest films.

Case 99: I.N. (02–19–73), a 24-year-old gravida 3, para 2, aborta 1, had a normal term delivery in October, 1956. In October, 1958, 2 years later, she developed vaginal bleeding; Curettage showed decidual tissue, and biopsy of a nodule in the vagina was diagnosed as choriocarcinoma. She was admitted to NIH on October 19, 1958; the HCG titer was about 200,000 units, and a chest x-ray showed bilateral pulmonary densities interpreted as being consistent with either bronchopneumonia or metastatic lesions. She received four courses of methotrexate; the HCG titer declined promptly to 200–500 units, and the chest lesions gradually cleared, and finally disappeared in November, 1959. In January, 1960, the HCG titer was 10–50 units. The patient was followed and remained free from evidence of trophoblastic disease through February, 1964, 7 years and 4 months after delivery. She delivered a healthly male infant on August 15, 1962, over 3 years after her discharge from NIH.

This case is classified as "probable" choriocarcinoma because the histopathological diagnosis rests on biopsy of a vaginal nodule which, although strongly suggestive of choriocarcinoma, particularly in the clinical context in which it was taken, was not sufficiently well preserved to permit a definitive microscopical diagnosis. The problem is similar to that in case 98: infiltration of vaginal tissue by a neoplasm which is partly hemorrhagic and largely necrotic. Again, however, the clinical, endocrinological, and radiological features most strongly suggest choriocarcinoma.

Case 100: L.M. (02–26–17), a 42-year-old Negro gravida 5, para 2, aborta 2, mole 1, had the following sequence of pregnancies; term delivery in 1952, abortion at 3 months in 1953, hydatidiform mole in August, 1956, abortion at 10 weeks in November, 1957, and normal term delivery on September 25, 1958. Following the hydatiform mole in 1956, menses resumed normally, and Friedman tests were negative. At a routine postpartum examination in November, a nodule about 5×2 cm was found on the right vaginal wall; a frog test for pregnancy was negative at this time. Biopsy of the vaginal nodule was diagnosed as choriocarcinoma; she was admitted to NIH on December 4, 1958. The HCG titer was between 5,000 and 10,000 units; a chest x-ray revealed several nodular densities in the right lung field and a single nodule in the left lower lung field. After four courses of methotrexate, the hormone titer was 50–200 units, and the chest film showed partial regression of the nodules. She was discharged on March 15, 1959, with almost no visible lesions in the chest film, an HCG titer of < 200 units, and a small focus of induration at the site of the vaginal nodule. She was followed to December, 1964, slightly more than 6 years after the onset of her disease; there was no evidence of recurrent disease.

This case is classified as "probable" choriocarcinoma because the histopathological diagnosis depends on one slide of a biopsy from a vaginal nodule which, although strongly suggestive, is not conclusively diagnostic of choriocarcinoma. As in the previous cases in this group, the diagnosis of choriocarcinoma hinges partly on the clinical circumstances, but it is difficult to postulate any other lesion that would behave in this fashion.

Printed in the United States of America